Praise for *The Diet Detox*

"I've always believed that fitness begins in the kitchen, and Brooke's *Diet Detox* really simplifies how to stop dieting and upgrade your nutrition in just 10 simple steps."

> —Jorge Cruise, celebrity trainer and author of *Tiny and Full*

"*The Diet Detox* is a fantastic book that cuts out all the BS and gives readers exactly what they need to know to lose weight and get healthy for life!"

> —Dave Asprey, founder and CEO of Bulletproof

"If you really do hate the word 'diet,' this is the book for you. Brooke has put together an incredibly easy-to-follow guide to help weed through all the nutritional chaos and get back on track for good."

> —Jenna Wolfe, host of Fox Sports 1's *First Things First*

"Bravo to Brooke Alpert for taking the diet out of dieting! Her 10 simple rules are all we need for lasting weight loss and good health. As an internist, I'm thrilled for my patients to ditch the 'yo-yo' diet dead-end for healthy eating habits they can stick to. *The Diet Detox* is just what the doctor ordered!"

> —Holly L. Phillips, MD, author of *The Exhaustion Breakthrough*

The Diet Detox

The Diet Detox

*Why Your Diet Is Making You Fat
and What to Do About It*

Brooke Alpert, MS, RD, CDN

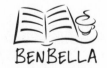

BenBella Books, Inc.
Dallas, TX

BenBella Books, Inc.
10440 N. Central Expressway, Suite 800
Dallas, TX 75231
www.benbellabooks.com
Send feedback to feedback@benbellabooks.com

Printed in the United States of America
10 9 8 7 6 5 4 3 2 1

Library of Congress Cataloging-in-Publication Data:
Names: Alpert, Brooke, author.
Title: The diet detox : why your diet is making you fat and what to do about it : 10 simple rules to help you stop dieting, start eating, and lose the weight for good / Brooke Alpert, MS, RD, CDN.
Description: Dallas, TX : BenBella Books, Inc., [2018] | Includes bibliographical references and index.
Identifiers: LCCN 2017042965 (print) | LCCN 2017047025 (ebook) | ISBN 9781944648992 (electronic) | ISBN 9781944648923 (trade cloth : alk. paper)
Subjects: LCSH: Reducing diets. | Reducing diets--Recipes. | Weight loss. | Detoxification (Health)
Classification: LCC RM222.2 (ebook) | LCC RM222.2 .A3956 2018 (print) | DDC 613.2/5--dc23
LC record available at https://lccn.loc.gov/2017042965

Editing by Leah Wilson and Rachel Holtzman
Copyediting by Jennifer Brett Greenstein
Proofreading by Michael Fedison and Greg Teague
Indexing by Jigsaw Information
Text design and composition by Publishers' Design and Production Services, Inc.
Front cover design by Ty Nowicki
Jacket design by Sarah Avinger
Printed by Lake Book Manufacturing

Distributed to the trade by Two Rivers Distribution, an Ingram brand
www.tworiversdistribution.com

Special discounts for bulk sales (minimum of 25 copies) are available. Please contact Aida Herrera at aida@benbellabooks.com.

To anyone who has ever said, "The diet starts Monday."

Contents

A Letter to the Reader

S o you've decided to buy a diet book. It's a fabulous invest-
ment, but I want to warn you before you read any further that this
isn't going to be your *typical* diet book. There's a way to eat that's going
to make you feel good and help you achieve your goals, and then there's
everything else. What you are going to get from me is the honest truth
about how to finally lose the weight that's been holding you back. Dieting
is hard work; I've seen it in my private nutrition counseling and weight
loss practice for the last decade. But it's not about willpower—it's about
being smart with what and how you eat. If you want to change the way
you look and feel, then you're going to have to permanently change the way
you look at food and dieting. It's not rocket science, and it doesn't need to
be overly complicated or restrictive—at the end of the day, it's just food.

Leave the diets you've done in the past in the past. Let those fad
moments go; let go of the 30 days of healthy eating you committed to only
to overindulge in pizza, ice cream, or whatever your guilty pleasure is.
Let go of the exhausting weight loss, weight gain, weight loss cycle. And
instead, let's do this! I've made it as easy as possible to make long-lasting
positive changes. In exchange, what I'm asking of you is simple: do my
one-week jump-start program and then follow my 10 rules. You might
have heard of versions of them before—you might even have tried some
of them before. But you've never put them all together like this.

What I'm offering in *The Diet Detox* is the real deal. It's the same
guidance I give my clients, and it's the same advice I give my friends. In
fact, I've even incorporated a lot of their questions and my honest answers
throughout the chapters. This is the way I speak in my own personal life:
clear and to the point. I'm going to give you some of the tools I use in
my practice for shaping the way you eat, but more important, I'm going

to give you the 10 rules for how you should be eating for the rest of your life. Reading this book and following the rules every day is the only way to lose the weight and keep it off for good.

In health and honesty,
Brooke

The 10 Rules

E VERY CLIENT who comes to my private practice, B Nutritious in New York City, leaves his or her first session with a list of 10 rules, or goals to work on. I charge a huge amount of money for this, but I'm giving it to you here for the price of this book. What I tell my clients—and what I consistently remind them of—is that even though these rules or goals seem small or like common sense, they add up to a massive diet overhaul. The same 10 rules form the backbone of this book, and they will get you exactly where you want to go with your weight and health. Note that there's no kitschy shtick here, nothing trendy, and definitely nothing extreme. That's because any diet worth your time shouldn't have an expiration date. It's a lifestyle, regardless of how much I hate that cliché expression. These are the fundamentals that I use in my practice with every client at B Nutritious. There are just 10 things you need to be doing right now, with no negotiating. This is how to eat and how to live a healthy life in just 10 steps. To get started, look over the list on the next page, head to the one-week Kick-Starter on page 17, and then start reading the chapters to see how to incorporate these 10 rules into your life from now on.

1. Eat Protein and Fiber at Every Meal

What I find so great about this rule is that it gives you a very clear and simple way to look at your plate. Is there a protein source? Check. Is there a fiber source? Check. Both protein and fiber (and fat: see Rule #4) do some incredible things. First, they are both very satiating, so your meal feels satisfyingly filling. A spicy lemonade à la Master Cleanse certainly can't do that. Protein and fiber also help slow down the absorption of sugar into your bloodstream. This is because they take longer to digest,

THE RULES

1. **Eat Protein and Fiber at Every Meal**

2. **Check Your Starches**

3. **Clock Your Meals**

4. **Eat Fat**

5. **Watch the Sugar**

6. **Indulge Intentionally**

7. **Supplement Smartly**

8. **Get Some Sleep**

9. **Drink Water**

10. **Exercise**

allowing your blood sugar levels to remain more stable, which leads your weight and energy levels to remain stable.

2. Check Your Starches

This isn't a low-carb diet. Well, actually, it's not a diet at all, but you get the idea. While I'm not recommending that you keep track of your carb intake, you do need to be aware of how many *starches* you eat per day. There are a few reasons for this: First, starches are the easiest foods to overeat—how many people normally eat a half cup of pasta? Not me! Second, the majority of starches (think the bready stuff) are high in sugar, even if they're savory foods, which makes overeating starches the number one way to put on weight. Omitting them altogether sets you up to fail, but eating them in a controlled way will not only help you lose weight but also prevent you from feeling deprived.

"I have been dieting and following the Diet Detox seriously for nine months. In that time, I have lost an incredible amount of weight; I never dreamed this was possible. The Diet Detox offers a food algorithm with endless options, but in a simple form to eliminate any confusion. Thanks to the Diet Detox, I've never felt so content about my weight or my appetite."

—Phil. G., lawyer

3. Clock Your Meals

The ultimate goal in permanent weight loss and good health is to keep your blood sugar and your energy levels stable. Waiting too long between having meals or snacks sets you up to fail. Period. Most poor food choices are made because you're too hungry to think straight—prevent that from happening by eating regularly. That's why I want you to have a meal or a snack every 4 hours. You don't need to set an alarm to keep you on an exact, to-the-minute schedule, but you should make sure you are eating regularly. Note: This is not the same as grazing all day. There must be a start and a finish to every meal or snack—otherwise you might end up eating like a cow that grazes on grass all day. Plus, I want you to be finished with eating a couple of hours before you go to sleep. Ideally you're leaving 12 to 14 hours between your dinner and your breakfast the next morning.

4. Eat Fat

Fat-free is so nineties. Move on to the new millennium and realize that fat is *not* the enemy but actually your weight loss friend. When you remove fat from a food product (cookies, dairy, anything), most of the time you end up with higher sugar levels. That's no good. Fat keeps you full; slows down the absorption of sugar, like your friends' protein and fiber do; helps you absorb major nutrients from your food, like vitamins A, E, D, and K; regulates your hormones; and keeps your brain functioning optimally. And let's be honest, it tastes good. This is a huge deal, because when a food is intrinsically satisfying, we need less of it to feel satisfied. No more of that almost-blue skim milk for you!

5. Watch the Sugar

I'm known as the anti-sugar nutritionist. I literally wrote the book on sugar and the havoc it can wreak on your body. Cliff's Notes version: Sugar makes you fat and ages you prematurely. There's nothing good here. Natural sugars found in fruits get a slight pass as long as they are portion controlled, but there are no freebies in this nondiet diet, aside from green veggies. Artificial sweeteners are an absolute no—even the organic ones. Read more in chapter four about the nonnegotiables. There is a time and a place for a slice of cake or a scoop of ice cream—check out Rule #6 for more on that. In the meantime, stop making your morning coffee a milk shake, and don't try to tell me you don't have a sweet tooth—I see that sugar in your white bread!

6. Indulge Intentionally

I'm not unrealistic. I know that in life there are moments when you just gotta have a bagel or doughnut, or whatever your heart desires (within reason here, people). It just needs to be *intentional*. When you make a deliberate decision to eat a food that would normally be considered unhealthy, you're allowing yourself to eat this indulgence in a controlled manner. In contrast, if you say you will never again eat a scoop of ice cream, then you set yourself up to be a whole pint deep by the end of the week. By planning for these intentional indulgences, we eliminate the guilt that gets associated with these foods and that can lead to overeating. I say it regularly in my practice: guilt is the number one cause of weight gain. An intentional indulgence is literally how to have cake and eat it too.

7. Supplement Smartly

My ultimate goal would be for people to get all the nutrition they need from their food. That would be ideal. Except it's not possible, because it's hard to keep up with the body's demands even with a great diet. But today's multivitamins are antiquated. They don't focus enough on what we really need, and they don't focus on the best time of day to absorb nutrients. Later in this book I'll break down the supplements you will actually benefit from into two categories: the "essential" ones, which almost everyone needs to take daily, and the "bonus" ones, which can help you optimize your health, your energy levels, and your optimal weight.

"Over the past few years, I have attempted countless diets and spent hours in the gym. Nothing had a lasting effect. I would lose weight and gain it right back. The cycle repeated itself over and over again. It was not until I tried the Diet Detox that I lost the weight I had been holding onto for so long and, more important, kept it off. The Diet Detox is simple and doable. The success I achieved with the Diet Detox awoke the determination and focus that I needed to start reaching my goals."

—B.D., stay-at-home mom

8. Get Some Sleep

Setting yourself up for success means starting the day right. And while I'm obviously a fan of breakfast (see Rule #3), if you aren't regularly getting an adequate amount of sleep, you are starting every day with a major deficit. When we don't get enough sleep (typically 7 to 8 hours a night), our hormones shift and our bodies literally tell us to eat more. Unfortunately, we're getting told not to eat a kale salad but to have a quick, sugary fix that gives our bodies a jolt of energy. Thus begins the vicious cycle of sugar highs and sugar lows. In chapter four, I'll describe what counts as good sleep and how to get more of it.

9. Drink Water

Water should be your primary beverage. Not a sports drink, not coffee, not coconut water, but free ol' water. So often, thirst is mistaken for hunger, and dehydration leads us to fatigue, making us want to reach for something sweet for a pick-me-up. This can become a vicious cycle. Instead, get a cute water bottle, fill it up in the morning, and finish it by the end of the day. Aim for at least 1.5 liters a day. The benefits include clearer skin, more energy, controlled hunger, weight loss, and pee breaks. That last one may not be the best benefit, but at least it'll get you moving a little more.

10. Exercise

Diet takes the weight off, but exercise helps keep it off. If you want to keep this weight off for good and to continue to lose weight, then you have to move, ideally for 30 minutes a day. Some workouts are better than others—high-intensity interval training is the best, but just get moving. Don't allow more than two days in a row without some type of movement happening!

These rules aren't super-tough to follow, but as I say to my clients, when you put them all together, you are completely changing the way you eat and live. I'm also a realist, so throughout this book you'll see how to incorporate these rules into your *real* daily life, including special occasions, events, trips, or anything that's gotten in your way in the past. I've basically put your new eating plan on a silver platter for you!

Chapter 1

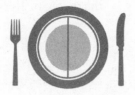

Diet Takedown

A CCORDING TO *Merriam-Webster's Collegiate Dictionary*, the definition of *diet* is:

1. a. food and drink regularly provided or consumed
   b. habitual nourishment
   c. the kind and amount of food prescribed for a person or animal for a special reason
   d. a regimen of eating and drinking sparingly so as to reduce one's weight

In all my research, I've never found anything that says a diet means drinking only lemon water for five days, consuming frozen pre-packaged meals, counting every food as a specific point, or eating like people did during a specific time in history. How have we managed to turn a simple word like *diet* into a dirty word? And how have we moved so far from eating in a way that makes sense that we are now constantly trying out these bizarre and random programs that don't work? Actually, maybe I shouldn't complain about this. Over 50 percent of my female clients are Weight Watchers dropouts. These diets are actually feeding my business, so I thank you, (insert any mass diet name here).

There are tons of programs out there; in fact, I've even created one for dealing with sugar addiction, but all of them—including mine—have an expiration date. Therein lies the problem. The diets we're trying are setting us up for failure. How many times did you start one only to stop it and then gain more weight back than you lost? How many times have you uttered to yourself, "The diet starts on Monday"? Why are we doing this to Monday almost every week? Monday is hard enough without making it a day to start following an unreasonable diet! Not to mention what we do to poor Sunday. This day of rest has turned into everyone's last meal. People eat extra poorly because the next day they are going to finally start eating better. So Sunday is loaded with extra goodies, Monday starts with a great intention, and then by Wednesday, you've fallen off the wagon. This is a terrible cycle that I see over and over again. What you need to do is eat the right way for life. Every single day. The Diet Detox is setting you up for a lifetime of healthy eating. You should be eating food, not calories, not points, not something that gets rehydrated to potentially resemble something edible. Real food that tastes good and that does something beneficial for your body. There should be flexibility to allow you to indulge without setting you up for failure. If you're doing it right, then you won't ever need to utter the words "I just blew my diet."

Research even supports that dieting can actually lead to weight gain. A 2013 study published in *Frontiers in Psychology* that reviewed 25 *other* studies about restrictive eating for weight loss showed that dieting significantly predicted future weight gain. In other words, these researchers found evidence that simply dieting led to almost certain weight gain. Why is this? The yo-yo factor is a big one—you lose some, you gain some more, it's then harder to lose again, and the cycle continues. Studies have now shown that this is because weight gain after weight loss leads to major changes in your gut and your microbiome (the bacteria that's found in your GI system). Basically each time you lose weight and then gain it back, the ratio of your so-called "skinny" bacteria to your "fat" bacteria gets skewed. Each yo-yo diet leaves your gut with more of the fat-producing bacteria, making it even harder for you to lose weight. This is one reason why probiotic use and gut health are so important, and why I'll be talking more about them in chapter four. Other studies have shown that perhaps our bodies aren't evolved enough to deal with weight loss that's achieved in an unhealthy way, or that our brains prevent our bodies from losing weight in order to protect ourselves from starvation. Regardless of the reasoning, traditional dieting sets you up for failure, weight gain, and a true hatred of Monday.

Truth: Not every diet out there is terrible. Some are decent or have done positive things for the nutrition world. Some have interesting ideas. But for the most part, diets are bunk. What else is wrong with them? Take a look at my diet takedown.

Let's get ready to rumble!

Master Cleanse

I feel like I shouldn't even need to write about this one—come on, people! Living on a lemon juice, cayenne pepper, and maple syrup concoction is no way to get through life, even for the 10 days that it's recommended. Not only are you physically depleted and lacking in energy because, hello, you're not eating, but you lose muscle

Q. Should I do a cleanse?

A. I get asked this all the time, and while I think it is always best to learn from your own mistakes, let me prevent you from wasting your time, money, and toilet paper. Most cleanses are super-restrictive and leave you hungry. This is just another setup for yo-yo dieting and the start-stop weight loss that makes it more and more difficult to reach your ideal weight. Let's also not forget that our bodies are not like a dirty carpet that needs regular cleaning. Our liver, kidneys, skin, and othwer organs are constantly doing that work. If you feel like you need a push, that is the beauty of my one-week Kick-Starter program. Opt for that instead.

mass, spend too much time in the bathroom, and totally sabotage any redeeming healthy relationship you might have had with food. While I've seen plenty of people lose weight in the few days they stay on the Master Cleanse, everyone I know who has done it has gained the weight back plus a few pounds. Even worse, many end up having a food binge afterwards because of the huge amount of deprivation.

Juice Cleanses

My issues with juicing are similar to my issues with the Master Cleanse. No real food makes people unhappy and hungry. Don't get me wrong, I love a good green juice with one small piece of fruit plus a lemon in it, but juicing all day—for multiple days—is another way to set yourself up for failure. Many juices are super-high in sugar, and when you're done with the cleanse, then what? I have seen so many people do a juice cleanse for three days and then go for pizza. They're totally missing the point. Such restriction leads to poor choices, and it's not teaching you any sustainable lessons about health or eating.

Weight Watchers

I'm not joking when I say I owe Weight Watchers a thank-you note. The stories from my former Weight Watchers clients usually go like this: they lose weight to start, then either plateau and can't seem to lose any more weight, or hit their goal weight but can't maintain it. I do like that there is a place for all foods in the program, and the idea of figuring out how to fit in that cookie is a smart life lesson, but at the end of the day, food isn't numbers. We don't eat points; we eat food. When we get so removed from understanding what our plate should look like, we lose our way and gain weight. And not all food is created equal—you can hit your numbers by eating just fat-free, sugar-free ice cream and other nutritionally empty foods. But the number you won't hit is the one you want to see on the scale.

Jenny Craig

I had a client who was a big Jenny Craig user. She loved the convenience of the frozen food and had her freezer stocked with the meals. Great, right? Nope—she felt terrible. Not only was she not losing weight, but she also had skin issues and low energy. By the time she came to me, she had been eating frozen meals for months. And she discovered that these meals are often packed with ingredients that aren't exactly whole foods. I love convenience, but the food also has to be healthy. There is no substitute for real food, made with real ingredients.

Paleo

My answer here might surprise you: I don't think this diet program is half-bad. I like that its recommendations prompted more conversations about the quality of our meat, fish, and other animal products. Most people weren't considering grass-fed and organic meat and poultry before the Paleo diet took off. One small issue I have with this plan is that it eschews some healthy although not totally necessary foods like whole grains and beans. But my biggest problem is that the allowances aren't "real-life" enough. Meaning, unless it's a Paleo-style cupcake, there isn't room to have a slice of cake. I've seen many people struggle with this diet because there's so little wiggle room, and after one indulgence they're typically thrown off track. The Whole30 is a subset of the Paleo diet that I don't mind, but it's a 30-day plan. It's meant to be a diet reset of sorts, and in this regard it is similar to the Kick-Starter program in this book, but the Whole30 is so limiting that I see it having a yo-yo effect on people.

"After a few months of sticking to the Diet Detox, I don't think I'm on a diet anymore. I'm just eating normally, but it's a different 'normally' than a few months ago. Feeling great has been the ultimate reward, and sensible eating is now a part of my everyday practice thanks to the easy Diet Detox rules! I don't see an end in sight."

—J.T., therapist

Low-Carb

There are a bunch of different diet plans out there that people refer to as some sort of low-carbohydrate diet. My biggest problem with this type of diet plan is that people are usually misinformed about it. I often get new clients who say they follow a low-carb diet, but when we go through what they eat every day, I see that their diet is filled with carbohydrates. Fruit, dairy, and vegetables all contain carbohydrates. So what these clients are actually doing is watching their starches (breads, pastas, grains, and so on). While I support that (see Rule #2), I have found that when people limit an entire food group, they set themselves up for failure.

"My grueling work hours and stress led me to opt for convenience foods rather than home-cooked healthy foods. My diet consisted of ready-made, precooked meals. Over time I grew heavier and soon I was 40 pounds overweight—I needed to take control of my health. The Diet Detox helped me gain control over my health. I needed something simple that could work with my busy lifestyle. Because the Diet Detox was so simple to understand, I was able to set myself up for long-term success. I now have a better understanding of the fundamental food groups that are essential for mindful eating."

—Carrie D., medical student

Case Study: Lindsay

Lindsay came to me shortly after I opened my practice. She had come to me on the advice of her trainer, who had seen her weight go up and down about five times. Lindsay had tried every diet out there and was struggling with a sort of diet overload. She had just finished four months of Jenny Craig and had been eating only frozen prepared foods. But when she went to a restaurant, she would go crazy and completely overeat. This poor woman had literally forgotten how to eat normally after years of trying out different diets. When she wasn't trying out a new diet, she was gaining weight. Each time she put on weight, she'd put on more weight than she had gained previously, which meant that she would have even more weight to lose the next time she dieted. Her pattern was beyond unhealthy.

When we first met in my office, she was ready to go on a crazy restrictive diet, but after hearing her diet history, I gave her a modified plan. I allowed her two starches a day and two indulgences a week, and asked her to give me a month with weekly visits. These weekly visits were important because I knew her weight loss would be a little on the slow side, even though it would ultimately be slow and steady. The visits would provide her with the pep talks she needed to keep doing what she was doing. By the end of the first month she was down 5 pounds. That was not a lot, especially for four weeks, but it was enough to keep her going. My goal was to show her that she could lose weight and get to a healthy number by eating the right way instead of following this crazy yo-yo crash course she had been on. Each session I'd ask her if she was hungry, craving anything, or feeling like she was struggling with eating like this. Every time her response was, "I could eat like this for the rest of my life."

After three months she was down almost 20 pounds! And by five months she was at her goal weight—something she hadn't seen for longer than a week at a time during each of her diet attempts. Lindsay still checks in with me every now and again, but it's almost 10 years later and she is still at her goal weight, with no expiration date in sight.

Chapter 2

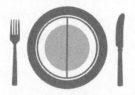

Give Me One Week:
The Kick-Starter

I LOVE READING OTHER DIET BOOKS. I sometimes learn something new, but usually I get to have a good laugh or be totally shocked. The thing that infuriates me the most is having to read pages and pages without actually understanding *what the plan is*. So let's put it right here, front and center. What is this new lifestyle really about? Sure, you have the 10 rules, but exactly what do you eat next?

Even though this is the anti-diet diet, I think it's still important to take a break from your regular eating and living habits in order to form new habits. So before we get started with your new way of eating for life, I'm asking you to give me one week. Just seven days of your undivided attention and appetite to rein things in, start from zero, and build from there. This one-week Kick-Starter will help lay the foundation for a lifetime of healthy eating. And yes, you might drop a few pounds while you're at it.

This week will take the most important components of the 10 rules and break them down into the simplest concepts of how to

> *"Wow! I lost 5 pounds (5!) in one week, and I wasn't hungry. To put the number in perspective, I'm 5 feet 3 inches and in pretty good shape, and I already eat healthy, whole foods. This jump start was amazing, and I'm on board to make a lifetime eating change."*
>
> —L.K., entrepreneur

Do You Need Some Help?

If you need extra motivation to start this new program, I recommend adding Provance by Rebody or Fit Kick by Twinlab to your Kick-Starter. They both contain an herbal blend called Slimvance that will help your blood sugar stay steady and help control your hunger hormones. Read more about it and the recommended dosage in chapter four.

eat. Because even though all 10 rules are important, sometimes even 10 rules are too many for just getting started.

During this time, I'm going to be a little more strict with you than usual. I'll be limiting the options for your proteins, fibers, and starches. This is not to be mean but to make the transition easier for you. Studies have shown that when there are fewer options to chose from, you're less likely to take a misstep. Think of this as the Steve Jobs uniform for meal planning. Normally I like variety—and that's exactly what you'll get with the Diet Detox program—but for one week, the Kick-Starter is ideal. So let's keep this short and sweet. You'll find a full list of Kick-Starter-approved foods—and their recommended serving sizes—on page 17.

I'm also a fan of using supplements to round out your nutrition and help you lose weight, and I'll go into much more detail in chapter four. But for getting started, I'll have you stick with just my favorite fiber supplement, FibeHER by Reserveage. Take FibeHER every morning before breakfast to help you get in some extra fiber—which is beneficial because it helps stabilize your blood sugar levels, which in turn helps control your

Are You Truly Hungry?

It's easy to get confused about what our body is actually telling us when it comes to hunger, especially when we're trying to adapt to a new way of eating. Even though I'm not touting deprivation here, see if you can get to the root of why you're feeling hungry. If you've just eaten yet still feel hungry, shake things up. Go to a different room, start a different project at work, drink more water, call a friend, or scroll through Facebook, for Pete's sake. It's often mind games, thirst, and sugar cravings that have us reaching for more when we truly don't need anything else to eat. However, if you really do feel true hunger, go ahead and eat more, but stick to the options that I've offered on page 17. If those don't appeal to you, that's a great way to tell if your body is just faking you out.

cravings and your weight. It also contains protein to keep you feeling full and satisfied from the start of the day.

Here is the plan:

1. Every morning before breakfast, take 1 scoop (14.8 grams) FibeHER fiber supplement with an 8-ounce glass of water.
2. Every meal needs to have a serving of protein and a serving of fiber (P & F). Each snack should include protein and/or fiber. You can pick one of the three options from the protein category and one of the fiber options (see the meal guidelines on page 13). If you are still hungry, you may have an additional fiber.
3. Add fat to your protein or fiber in every meal. Cook your eggs in grass-fed butter or coconut oil. Use olive oil on your salad or sauté your vegetables in ghee. Add half of an avocado to any meal. Note: Dairy and nut products already contain fat, so they'll do double duty as fat and protein. If you have a full-fat Greek yogurt for breakfast, then you don't have to think about fat—it's already included.
4. You are allotted only one serving of starch (S) per day. Choose one of the three options on page 13 at lunch or at dinner. I recommend saving your starch for lunch or dinner to keep your blood sugar levels even and help you sleep better.
5. Try to follow the serving sizes I recommend on page 17, but do not go hungry! Remember, this isn't about deprivation; it's about getting back on track. If you're truly hungry and you're not just bored or thirsty, add more of the protein or fiber options to your meal or snack. But before you do, read "Are You Truly Hungry?" on page 10.

> *"The one-week Kick-Starter will definitely influence the way I eat. I've been trying to be 'good' for ages. Being 'good' (restricting myself) rarely translated into successful weight loss, though. This program didn't feel like a diet—I feel great!"*
>
> —Jenny D, marketing manager

Pro Fat

Don't skimp on the fat, ever. Trust me on this one, especially for this week. Fat will keep you fuller, more satisfied, and less likely to pick a fight with your spouse.

6. No alcohol. It's one week—don't complain.

7. Drink a minimum of around 2 liters or 64 ounces of water a day. Add lemon or lime for flavor. Unsweetened tea is also fine, as is coffee, but limit it to 2 cups a day with ¼ cup of milk or a nondairy alternative. No sugar, please!

8. Aim to drink 1 to 2 cups of dandelion root tea per day (see page 197). Dandelion is a lot more than a weed. Tea made from its roots can boost weight loss, improve digestion, and regulate blood sugar levels, which makes it the perfect addition to this one-week program and to your diet afterwards. It's also caffeine-free, so feel free to drink it any time of day. My favorite brand is Alvita, which is both organic and high quality.

9. Need something sweet? You can have 1 ounce of good-quality dark chocolate a day. For the Kick-Starter program it must be at least 80 percent cocoa.

"I've tried almost every diet, most of them successfully, but lately even though I know what I'm supposed to do, I have a hard time sticking to a plan. Further complicating things, I'm a working mother of two young children, and I travel frequently for work. The simple rules of this diet helped me stay on track and full. The most important lesson for me is including healthy fat in my snacks and making sure I have these on hand. The one-week Kick-Starter was a great way to get my eating on track. Now that I'm following the 10 rules from the Diet Detox, I'm confident that I will see further success and will not need another diet again."

—R. Stone, creative director

What to Read

Ignore the nutrition label and go straight to the ingredient list. Make sure that there is no added sugar in your dressings, sauces, and condiments.

Meal Guidelines (see page 17 for serving sizes)

Pre-breakfast

FibeHER fiber supplement

Breakfast

Protein *(pick one):* Eggs, full-fat yogurt, nut butter

Fiber *(pick one):* Berries, spinach, apple

Lunch

Protein *(pick one):* Sliced turkey, canned/jarred tuna, chicken

Fiber *(pick one):* Mixed greens, cucumbers, peppers

Starch *(pick one):* Multigrain bread, rice, whole-wheat wrap

Add a fat (see below)

Snack

Protein *(pick one):* Nuts, full-fat yogurt, hummus

Fiber *(pick one):* Berries, carrots, apple

Dinner

Protein *(pick one):* Fish, chicken, beef

Fiber *(pick one):* Mixed greens, cauliflower, broccoli

Starch *(if you didn't eat a starch at lunch, pick one):* Rice, quinoa, sweet potato

Add a fat (see below)

Suggested Fats to Be Used in Every Meal

Olive oil, coconut oil, avocado, guacamole, butter (ideally grass-fed), ghee. Note that full-fat yogurt, nut butters, eggs, and nuts also count as fats.

Condiments and Seasonings

Salt, pepper, mustard (no sugar added), balsamic vinegar, lemon, lime, tomato sauce (no sugar added), salsa (no sugar added), onions, garlic, herbs and spices, tamari

"This diet was completely manageable and has kick-started what I hope is a change in lifestyle. I had a baby seven months ago and it has been hard getting rid of the belly after my C-section. My stomach definitely flattened and I feel like I am on my way to getting my body back. I am also feeding my child healthy foods, and I want to set a good example with what I am eating."

—Jayme, school counselor

This week doesn't include any desserts, or "intentional indulgences" as I call them. I realize that Rule #6 is often my clients' favorite part of my diet plan. And yes, it's exciting to be able to find room on your plate for whatever you're honestly craving and to eat it guilt-free. But be honest with yourself—have you indulged lately? Did you indulge last night, knowing you were about to start a new diet plan today? Was this past Sunday your last hurrah? Let's come clean with one another: there are no indulgences this week because if you weren't overindulging to begin with, you wouldn't have picked up this book!

While I want to keep you away from the need to be on and off a diet, every so often we all need a push to get back on track. Perhaps you need a push to lose weight for a fancy event or a reunion, or maybe you need one to help you make it past a weight loss plateau. This week can be that for you. Let this week be your reminder of what clean eating really is and what it feels like to be saying no to desserts (aside from 1 ounce of dark chocolate a day—which isn't too shabby!), and then follow the 10 rules to start eating the right way for the rest of your life. Let this be the last time you start a diet.

#makeearlybirdcool

If you can, try not to eat dinner later than 7:00 PM. I'm trying to make the early-bird special cool—can we hashtag that? #makeearlybirdcool. I'll discuss this in more detail later in the book, but it's a great habit to start now, not just for weight loss but for better sleep.

One Week at a Glance

Monday

Pre-breakfast: FibeHER fiber supplement

Breakfast: Scrambled eggs with spinach and salsa

Lunch: Mixed greens and cucumbers with tuna, lemon, olive oil, and half an avocado

Snack: Yogurt with berries

Dinner: Filet mignon with sautéed broccoli and quinoa

Tuesday

Pre-breakfast: FibeHER fiber supplement

Breakfast: Sliced apple with almond butter

Lunch: Whole-wheat wrap with sliced turkey, mustard, cucumber, and guacamole

Snack: Hummus with baby carrots

Dinner: Roasted chicken with cauliflower rice

Wednesday

Pre-breakfast: FibeHER fiber supplement

Breakfast: Yogurt with berries

Lunch: Lettuce wrap with grilled chicken, roasted red peppers, and olive oil and balsamic vinegar dressing

Snack: Apple and almonds

Dinner: Broiled salmon, rice, and a side salad with olive oil and balsamic vinegar dressing

Thursday

Pre-breakfast: FibeHER fiber supplement

Breakfast: Sliced hard-boiled eggs, half an avocado, and an apple

Lunch: Open-faced turkey sandwich with lettuce and cucumbers on multigrain bread

Snack: Hummus with baby carrots

Dinner: Hamburger patty on a bed of lettuce with salsa and a side of sautéed broccoli

Friday

Pre-breakfast: FibeHER fiber supplement

Breakfast: Sliced apple with almond butter

Lunch: Mixed greens with grilled chicken, avocado, cucumbers, peppers, and olive oil and balsamic vinegar dressing

Snack: Yogurt with berries

Dinner: Shrimp with quinoa and sautéed cauliflower

Saturday

Pre-breakfast: FibeHER fiber supplement

Breakfast: Poached eggs over sautéed spinach with a side of mixed berries

Lunch: Turkey and cucumber stick roll-ups dipped in mustard

Snack: Sliced apple with almond butter

Dinner: Baked sweet potato with shredded chicken, avocado, and salsa with a side salad

Sunday

Pre-breakfast: FibeHER fiber supplement

Breakfast: Yogurt with sliced apples and berries

Lunch: Open-faced tuna sandwich on multigrain bread with vinegar-dressed cucumbers

Snack: Hummus with baby carrots

Dinner: Ground beef sautéed in tomato sauce with broccoli and a side of mixed greens with olive oil and balsamic vinegar dressing and avocado

Kick-Starter Program

Shopping List and Serving Sizes

Protein	*Serving Size*
Eggs (ideally organic)	2–3
Yogurt (full-fat)*	5–7 ounces
Nut butter (no sugar added)*	2 tablespoons
Sliced turkey	6 ounces
Canned/jarred tuna*	1 (5–7 ounce) can/jar
Chicken (white or dark meat)	6 ounces
Nuts (all kinds)	⅓ cup, 1½ ounces (varies based on nut)
Hummus*	2 tablespoons
Fish (wild or sustainably farmed)	6 ounces
Beef (grass-fed or organic)	6 ounces

Fiber	
Berries (any kind)	1 cup
Spinach	2 cups (raw)
Apple	1 medium
Mixed greens (any besides iceberg)*	2 cups
Cucumbers	1 medium
Peppers	1 cup
Carrots (raw or cooked)	1 cup
Cauliflower (raw or cooked)	1 cup
Broccoli (raw or cooked)	1 cup

Starch	
Multigrain bread*	1 slice
Rice	½ cup (cooked)
Tortilla/wrap*	1 wrap

*For items marked with an asterisk, see brands I love on page 19.

| Quinoa | ½ cup (cooked) |
| Sweet potato | 1 small or ½ large |

Fat

Olive oil	1 tablespoon
Coconut oil	1 tablespoon
Avocado	½ avocado
Guacamole	¼ cup
Butter (grass-fed)*	1 tablespoon
Ghee	1 tablespoon

Miscellaneous

Dandelion root tea*

Salt

Pepper

Mustard (no sugar added)

Balsamic vinegar

Lemons

Limes

Tomato sauce (no sugar added)

Salsa (no sugar added)

Onions

Garlic

Herbs and spices (any)

Tamari

Brands I Love: Kick-Starter Edition

Yogurt: **Fage, Siggi's**

Nut butter: **NuttZo, Justin's, Barney Butter**

Canned/jarred tuna: **Tonnino** tuna fillets

Hummus: **Sabra**

Mixed greens: **Earthbound Farm**

Bread: **Food for Life Ezekiel 4:9** bread

Wraps: **La Tortilla Factory, Food for Life Ezekiel 4:9**

Butter: **Kerrygold**

Tea: **Alvita**

"The one-week plan was an excellent jump start to a committed and mindful eating plan to help curb cravings and get in touch with my hunger cues. As a dietitian and busy mom, I often find it hard to eat healthy and nutritiously when life is hectic. Time constraints and lack of planning make it hard to consistently choose healthy options throughout the day and therefore cause erratic eating. Using the guidelines and sample meal plans provided, I was able to shop and plan ahead for my daily meals and snacks. I became more mindful of my hunger and satiety cues and became more focused on sitting down to eat proper meals and snacks. After a few days of adjusting to the diet, I felt more energized and had fewer cravings for sugary and processed foods. I even had the energy to work out six days of the week! I would definitely recommend this diet to others."

—Jodi W., dietitian

---

*For a longer list of brands I love, see page 196.

Chapter 3

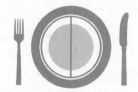

Let's Get Started

Y OU'VE DONE A WEEK, you've lost some weight, and you're feeling good—so what now? The next step is to follow my plan for life. That's the only thing that will get the weight to come off and stay off. But before you can get started, you have a little reading to do.

I gave you the one-week Kick-Starter for a little boost, perhaps as a bit of a shortcut to get your weight moving in the right direction and to motivate you to really clean up your act. But now it's time to put the 10 rules to work for good. If you follow the Diet Detox correctly, it can be a lifelong commitment—without being overly restrictive or making you "hangry" (a combination of hungry and angry—no joking matter!). I'm trying to empower you to make the right food choices with every single bite. What makes this so doable is that the right choice is not always kale or spinach but perhaps a bowl of spaghetti and a fudgy brownie. It's these kinds of allowances—along with a clear, concise, no-BS way of thinking about food—that will help you make a long-term commitment to this way of eating.

Let's take the 10 rules and put them into action now. In this chapter and the next chapters you'll read about each rule in great detail. (I had a word count commitment!) Also, it helps to know *why* you're doing the things you're doing.

RULES 1, 2, AND 3

1. Eat protein and fiber at every meal—just what it sounds like.
2. Check your starches—save them for lunch and/or dinner.
3. Clock your meals—eat every 4 hours (whether a meal or a snack); leave at least 12 to 14 hours between your dinner and the following breakfast.

Using just these rules every day, plus adding FibeHER and/or Provance by Rebody or Fit Kick by Twinlab, will have a major impact on how you feel. The following list shows how every day should look (remember that P is protein, F is fiber, and S is starch).

Cheat Sheet

For a more detailed list and serving sizes, check out page 17.

Protein: Eggs, chicken, turkey, beef, fish, shellfish, yogurt (all full-fat yogurts, but I especially vlike Greek or Icelandic), cottage cheese, cheese, beans, nuts, nut butter, hummus, chia seeds

Fiber: Fruits and vegetables (not including starchy vegetables like potatoes, sweet potatoes, butternut squash)

Starch: Potatoes, sweet potatoes, butternut squash, rice, quinoa, pasta, multigrain bread

Breakfast: P & F

Snack: P &/or F

Lunch: P & F + S

Snack: P &/or F

Dinner: P & F + S + end
    12 to 14 hours before your next meal

This is the plan. Every day. Yes, there are more nuances involved, but this is the basic idea. Each meal has a protein and a fiber. You can eat a starch or two with lunch and/or dinner. Once you've gotten through the one-week Kick-Starter program, this is your life for now on. Not just until bikini season is over, not just until 31 days are up, but forever. There's a place for chocolate (daily, see "Rule #4: Eat Fat" on page 55) and a place for cake or pizza (see "Rule #6: Indulge Intentionally" on page 68) but this is basically it. It's not complicated. It's not crazy restrictive. It's just how to eat to lose weight and keep it off, plain and simple. It's how to detox from all those crazy diets out there and simply eat for life. For more meal suggestions, check out page 143 for forty-five simple recipes that make the rules even easier to follow.

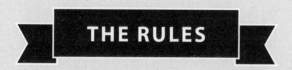

THE RULES

1. Eat protein and fiber at every meal.
2. Check your starches.
3. Clock your meals:
   a. Eat a meal or a snack every 4 hours.
   b. Make breakfast substantial and starch-free.
   c. Leave at least 12 to 14 hours between your dinner and the following breakfast.
4. Eat fat.
5. Watch the sugar.
6. Indulge intentionally.
7. Supplement smartly.
8. Get some sleep.
9. Drink water.
10. Exercise.

So how do these 10 rules work in our everyday lives? Let's talk this out. From the one-week Kick-Starter plan and the shortcut to the rules I gave you, you know how to combine a protein and a fiber, right? Let's turn this into a proper day.

You wake up, rested and refreshed (or like me, with two children jumping on you yelling for breakfast), and make some coffee—you use some full-fat milk and laugh at how you used to be addicted to artificial sweeteners. Time is a bit rushed, so you grab some hard-boiled eggs you prepared on Sunday (meal prep is always key!) and a couple of strawberries.

Breakfast, 7:00 AM: Coffee with milk, eggs (P), strawberries (F), water, FibeHER fiber supplement

You drive to work, get to the office, and check your email and possibly Facebook while you drink more water. As you check your calendar, you see that your scheduled lunch isn't until 1:00 PM and that's way too many hours to go between breakfast and lunch, so you need to figure out a snack.

Snack, 10:30 AM: Apple with a squeeze packet of almond butter, a cup or two of dandelion root tea

You drink some more water, have your conference calls, and continue to work. You check your pedometer or your Fitbit/Jawbone/whatever and see that you haven't moved too much today, so you go to the bathroom on the far side of the office. It's now time for lunch and you know that the restaurant you're going to for dinner has an awesome dessert, so you make sure lunch is clean to leave some room for an intentional indulgence later.

Lunch, 1:00 PM: Bowl of vegetable soup (F), half a turkey sandwich (P) (S)

More work and more water. You're prepared when you're stomach starts growling again, because when you grabbed lunch, you also grabbed a Greek yogurt for later.

Snack, 3:45 PM: Greek yogurt (P)

You wrap up work and head to dinner with friends at 6:15 PM. Your friends are still giving you a hard time about wanting to eat so early, but they're slowly getting on board here (#makeearlybirdcool).

Dinner, 6:15 PM: Arugula salad, steak frites—but no frites because that dessert is calling your name. Share a molten lava cake and enjoy every single bite!

"I have experimented with just about every diet, and I felt the Diet Detox was a gentle approach with dramatic results. It's really difficult for me to lose weight and to keep it off—but much to my surprise, I got through the first week without any problem and kept the weight off. What worked for me was the Kick-Starter week with strict choices so there was little room to make mistakes. Typically, when I pick a diet, it's a serious detox with food groups missing altogether and my body goes into shock! But on this plan, I learned to eat clean, balanced meals that left me feeling satisfied. By incorporating fat instead of starches in my meals and snacking only on whole foods, I stopped craving sugar during the day. I felt more focused and less sluggish, plus my skin never looked better. I would never go back to extreme diets—the Diet Detox provides both weight loss and long-term lifestyle habits that allow me to indulge in a dessert and not feel like I'm depriving myself. I would highly recommend the Diet Detox to anyone struggling to commit to a diet."

—Jen S., marketing manager

Say your goodbyes and head home, where you take your evening vitamins, relax, and get ready to do it all again tomorrow.

This is a pretty awesome day and I know that life doesn't always go that smoothly. Kids get sick, work gets crazy, cars break down, and so on. But if you can keep the main concepts of this plan going, then there is always room for a little bit of wiggle room. Being prepared is the best thing you can do to basically win at life, especially for anything that involves your diet. Preparing meals on Sunday for the week ahead is always great; cooking extra for dinner one night so you can bring your lunch to work the next day is also smart, both healthwise and financially. If you have more time and can be more ambitious with cooking and trying new recipes, that's great too! Taking those few minutes to think throughout the week allows you to set yourself up for success. It takes away most of your excuses because you have a healthy snack bar stashed in your desk or you always have almonds around. Most important, because you never feel deprived, you don't feel guilty, so you constantly make healthier and more consistent food choices. I say it all the time: guilt causes us to gain weight.

Let's look at another day on the Diet Detox and see how it works out:

Breakfast	*Time:* 6:30 AM
Greek yogurt with berries	(P) (F) S
Iced coffee	P F S
FibeHER fiber supplement	P (F) S
Snack	*Time:* 10:00 AM
Approved snack bar	
Lunch	*Time:* 12:30 PM
Salad from a salad bar—lettuce, celery, grilled chicken, apples, olive oil dressing	(P) (F) S
10 crackers (Mary's Gone Crackers)	P F (S)
Snack	*Time:* 3:00 PM
Hummus with baby carrots	
Dinner	*Time:* 6:30 PM
Frozen spinach	P (F) S
½ cup quinoa topped with tomato sauce and 2 fried eggs	(P) F (S)

This day looks really solid for eating. Granted, we're not talking about everything. Did this person exercise? Did she drink water? But you get the drift. She ate protein and fiber at every meal, ate about every 4 hours, included fat with all meals, and watched her starch portions. This day may seem slightly more restrictive than others, but remember she also had crackers with lunch and quinoa with dinner. She is never too hungry because she's eating so frequently, which makes the plan easier to stay on.

Now that we've looked at two really good days on the Diet Detox, let's take a look at some food diaries that I've received from clients and what I had to say about them.

This is a food diary a client recorded when she first started with me—let's call her Sam.

Breakfast		**Time: 7:30 AM**	
Special K with a banana and skim milk	P	F	S
Lunch		**Time: 1:00 PM**	
Turkey wrap	P	F	S
Diet soda	P	F	S
Dinner		**Time: 8:00 PM**	
Crackers while waiting for dinner	P	F	S
2 sushi rolls	P	F	S
2 glasses of wine	P	F	S
Snack		**Time: 9:30 PM**	
Handful of popcorn			

Now here is Sam's food diary with the marks I made when we had our session:

Breakfast	Time: 7:30 AM
Special K with a banana and skim milk *Where's the protein or legit fiber?*	P Ⓕ Ⓢ
Lunch	**Time: 1:00 PM**
Turkey wrap	Ⓟ Ⓕ S
Diet soda *So long between breakfast and lunch!*	P F Ⓢ
Dinner	**Time: 8:00 PM**
Crackers while waiting for dinner *No wonder she needed crackers while waiting for dinner–7 hours between meals is way too long!*	P F Ⓢ
2 sushi rolls	Ⓟ F Ⓢ
2 glasses of wine *Lots of starch, low on protein and fiber!*	P F S
Snack	**Time: 9:30 PM**
Handful of popcorn *Late-night snacking doesn't do anyone any good!*	

This food diary just brought me back a good 20 years as far as what we thought of as healthy eating. Sam thought she was a good, clean eater and didn't understand why she couldn't lose the 20 pounds that had crept up on her in the last decade. Introducing Sam to protein and fiber at every meal was a major step in the right direction. Changing up her meal timing was also really important. I don't know how some people go that long without a snack—maybe it's because I'm paid to talk and write about food all day, but my stomach literally starts growling as if it were an alarm clock when I'm approaching that 4-hour mark. Once we also checked Sam's starch portions and nixed the diet soda, we quickly saw some pretty major changes.

Let me show you what an ideal day in my life looks like, so you can see how I utilize all the rules at once. It's really how I try to live every single day whenever possible.

Wake up, 5:25 AM (thank you to my children, who believe 6:00 AM is way too late!): Lots of water

Breakfast, 6:45 AM: Black iced coffee, reheated frozen egg and spinach muffins

Workout, 8:30 AM: High-intensity interval training at my favorite studio, the Fhitting Room; tons of water

Snack, 10:30 AM: Apple dipped in almond butter

Lunch, 12:30 PM: Large chopped salad with avocado, grilled chicken, tons of veggies, extra-virgin olive oil, and lime juice; square of dark chocolate

Snack, 3:00 PM: Decaf latte, snack bar (mini Perfect Bar)

Dinner, 5:30 PM: Broiled salmon, broccoli, white rice

The more consistently these days happen for me, the more they tend to continue to happen. Tons of protein and fiber keep me feeling full, while eating regularly allows me to get to each meal or snack without losing any control because of hunger. This way of eating becomes second nature, and if there is a good indulgence to be had, it doesn't throw anything out of order. By the way, I don't believe dark chocolate is an indulgence. For me it's a necessity! As long as it's about 1 ounce a day, I'm happy for everyone to indulge daily in dark chocolate. The world might just be a better place if we all ate a little extra chocolate. Just make sure it's 70 percent cocoa or higher—otherwise it's a sugar bomb! During the Kick-Starter week, it must be 80 percent or higher.

So let's review again.

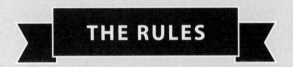

THE RULES

1. Eat protein and fiber at every meal.
2. Check your starches.
3. Clock your meals:
   a. Eat a meal or a snack every 4 hours.
   b. Make breakfast substantial and starch-free.
   c. Leave at least 12 to 14 hours between your dinner and the following breakfast.
4. Eat fat.
5. Watch the sugar.
6. Indulge intentionally.
7. Supplement smartly.
8. Get some sleep.
9. Drink water.
10. Exercise.

The most important rule, really, is #1: Eat protein and fiber at every meal. I delve into it a lot deeper in the next chapter, which explains why both of these nutrients are so crucial, but what I've found is that a clear-cut way of looking at their plate is the most effective tool I can create for my clients. You have become one of my clients by reading this book. If you can look at your plate and see that you have a healthy source of both protein and fiber for your meal, then there is not much more for you to have to think about. This doesn't need to be complicated—protein and fiber on your plate and you're good. The rest of it will come.

Chapter 4

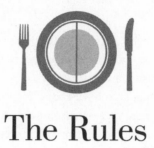

The Rules

Rule #1
P & F
Eat Protein and Fiber at Every Meal

As I mentioned earlier, every single client who walks into my office leaves his or her first session with a handful of goals to work on. Everyone's needs and health histories are different, but no matter what, the first directive for all my clients is to have P & F (protein and fiber) at each of their meals. I wanted to create a consistent objective that would help my clients determine if what they are eating is "correct." This makes it visually very clear and simple: if you can look at your plate and see a good source of protein and a good source of fiber, then you are good. Simple, right? P & F at every meal, please!

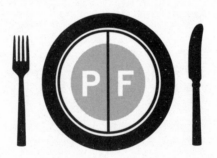

Protein

So what's the deal with protein? And why does it seem to be the cornerstone of every successful diet? For starters, you need to eat good-quality protein to keep your metabolism functioning and, equally as important, to keep your blood sugars stable. Diets high in protein have also been shown to be effective for reducing your appetite and your total caloric intake. A study published in the *American Journal of Clinical Nutrition* showed just that—it indicated that if you eat more protein, then you end up eating less overall. There's a connection between protein intake and meal satisfaction as well as satiety. Another study of overweight/obese men showed that when the 27 subjects followed a high-protein diet, they ate less at night, which helped control their appetite overall and increase their satiety, leading to weight loss. Protein consumption also helps create a process in the body called thermogenesis. Thermogenesis is basically the production of heat, particularly in the human body. This process helps the body burn energy. Since protein helps fuel thermogenesis, consuming protein leads to a greater caloric burn. Without enough protein in your body, your metabolism slows, it's harder to put on muscle mass, brain function and concentration problems occur, wounds don't heal, and mood issues can occur. As if regulating your metabolism wasn't enough of a reason to eat enough protein!

When I say "protein," I'm not asking you to eat a meat sandwich with meat as the bread and the filling, or to have your plate resemble a Lady Gaga dress. I'm asking you to make sure you have one serving of protein at each meal and that it is high quality, meaning that it's grass-fed, wild, or organic. While vegetarian foods can be great sources of protein (hello, chia seeds), the proteins in animal foods are superior. A protein is made out of something called amino acids. These amino acids can be found in vegetables and grains and even some fruits, but the best-quality amino acids come from animal sources. The amino acids in animal protein contain everything your body needs to build muscle mass, balance your hormones, support your brain, and prevent weight gain. So

So What Does a P & F Plate Look Like?

Breakfast

Omelet filled with spinach and Cheddar cheese (eggs–P, spinach–F)

Chia pudding with berries (chia–P, berries–F)

FibeHER fiber supplement

Lunch

Chopped romaine salad with chicken, cucumbers, and broccoli (chicken–P; romaine, cucumber, and broccoli–F)

Open-face sandwich on multigrain bread with turkey, mustard, and tomato and a small apple (turkey–P, tomato and apple–F, multigrain bread–S [for starch; see "Rule #2: Check Your Starches" on page 40])

Dinner

Sautéed shrimp over zucchini noodles with marinara sauce (shrimp–P, zucchini–F)

Steak with cauliflower and sweet potatoes (steak–P, cauliflower–F, sweet potatoes–S [for starch; see "Rule #2: Check Your Starches" on page 40])

Protein Options and Serving Sizes

Animal-Based

Always opt for organic, cage-free, grass-fed, or wild, if possible. For dairy, opt for full-fat, organic, or grass-fed.

2–3 eggs (whole)

6 ounces chicken or turkey

6 ounces red meat or pork

6 ounces fish or shellfish

5–7 ounces full-fat yogurt (unflavored)

1 ounce cheese

½ cup cottage cheese

¼ cup ricotta cheese

Plant-Based

6 ounces tofu (organic, non-GMO)

½ cup chickpeas, beans, lentils, or edamame

2 tablespoons hummus

2 tablespoons nut butter (no sugar added)

⅓ cup or 1½ oz nuts (all kinds)

2 tablespoons chia seeds

2 tablespoons hemp seeds

½ cup spirulina

unless my clients are vegans or vegetarians for religious or ethical reasons, I ask that they consider getting some of their protein from animal sources, even if they're just eggs.

In addition to its role in weight loss and weight maintenance, protein is important for many other factors in the body. Since proteins affect our neurotransmitter function and control the balance of our hormones—more specifically dopamine and serotonin—they have a big effect on our mood. Well-balanced dopamine levels help regulate emotional responses and can help prevent or reduce emotional eating—they basically allow you to walk away from that plate of cookies! Serotonin, a chemical messenger in the body, helps maintain an even-keeled mood and, just like with sugar in our blood, the more balanced our moods are, the better our food choices tend to be.

The amino acids found in protein also help keep our concentration levels up. This is one of the main reasons why breakfast should always contain a good-quality protein source. While this isn't a book about children, this rule definitely pertains to kids. If you want your children to be able to concentrate in school, skip the cold cereal (see "Making Breakfast Substantial—Ideally Without Starch" on page 50) and instead make sure they're getting a good-quality protein source. We adults are also expected to perform daily, and we depend on our brain function to help us focus and stay on the task at hand. Without the appropriate amino acids, our learning and our coordination skills will not be as sharp as they should be.

Case Study: Eden

I have a client named Eden who is fabulous and I really enjoy each session with her. Eden is a busy mom and is always on the run. She's a healthy eater for the most part, but when I looked at her food diary, I saw that her eating was all over the place. She had the best of intentions, but her diet was a total mishmash of foods. Eden never sat down for a meal until dinnertime, when she ate with her kids. Breakfast was on the go, lunch was on the run, snacking was all over the place, and then she'd be starving at dinner but didn't get why she overate at night!

She came to me looking to lose a few pounds and to get more energy, plus she just wanted to feel better overall. The first goal I worked on with Eden was the same one I work on with almost every client in my office: protein and fiber at every meal. Eden's breakfast was an apple or a bite of her daughter's leftovers before she left the house. Instead of eating an actual lunch, she would have small snacks all day and never eat protein and fiber together. She was almost resistant to the idea of proper and complete meals, saying that they would be too time-consuming to either prepare or eat.

When I saw she was overthinking the whole concept, I broke it down for her. First, I reminded her that we are all busy. People have kids, jobs, pets, and all kinds of responsibilities, but there is *always* time to take care of yourself in most situations. Second, she was already halfway there with most of her choices; she just needed to add the protein or the fiber. She was already eating an apple in the morning, so I told her to add some almond butter for protein (and a fat bonus!). She could have a yogurt and add some leftover fruit and/or chia seeds. I wasn't asking for a hot veggie-filled omelet, although that would be awesome too. I was just asking her to take an extra second to make sure there was a protein and a fiber at each meal. We worked on easy to-go lunches that wouldn't take a lot of prep work but would meet the requirements of protein and fiber; for example, she could add some sliced turkey to the carrots or pickles she was already eating. Obviously I would have loved to see some more greens in this meal, but I was going to take what I could get to prove to her that eating well wasn't so hard. Then once she got the protein and fiber down, I'd get pickier to help her make her meals even better. The whole goal for Eden was to have complete meals in order to feel better throughout the day and to set herself up for success so she wouldn't overeat at dinner. This seems like a small change, but it had a

big impact on her. At the next few sessions, Eden told me that she was feeling much more energetic and that she wasn't feeling deprived at all, even
though she was losing weight. Even better, Eden was no longer overdoing
it at dinner. That is a success in my book. Complete meals containing protein
and fiber are the ultimate way to set each meal up for success.

I am often asked about the connection between protein and heart
health. I focused on this issue in my previous book, *The Sugar Detox*, and
it's amazing how misled we have been. Sugar, not fat or protein, is the
biggest culprit for heart disease. All those fat-free foods that we ate in
the nineties were loaded with sugar, and that's what caused so many heart
health issues—not fat and cholesterol, which health experts at the time
suspected were the main culprits.

Despite all its benefits, not all protein is created equal. This is where
I often get some eye rolls from my clients, but it's important to make
smart choices about your protein sources. This is one of the parts of the
Paleo movement that I think is pretty awesome—it really opened up the
discussion of different protein sources and their quality; for example, those
on the Paleo diet opt for grass-fed beef whenever possible. Grass-fed beef
contains healthy saturated fats (you read that right; there is such a thing)
and a type of fat called conjugated linoleic acid (CLA), which has been
shown to cause fat *loss*. Many clinical trials have indicated the potential
of CLA to control body fat, reduce inflammation, and increase immune
functioning. The beef from grass-fed cows has 300 to 500 percent more
CLA content than that of grain-fed cows. Nutrition aside, most of the
time, grass-fed cows are raised in facilities that are more humane and
better for the environment, and they are not treated with hormones or
antibiotics. It's not hard to find grass-fed beef anymore, and it's becoming more affordable. If you can't find grass-fed beef, organic beef is a
suitable alternative. Another amazing protein source is wild fish, which
is filled with all the amino acids and tons of heart-healthy omega-3 fatty
acids. Farmed fish isn't the best option, as a lot of it is contaminated by
things we really don't want in our food supply, like antibiotics, pesti-
cides, and other toxins. Whenever possible, eat wild and sustainable fish.
There is a great website called Seafood Watch (www.seafoodwatch.org/

seafood-recommendations) that has tons of information about the best fish to eat for both health and the environment.

When in doubt about what kind of protein to buy, look for "grass-fed," "wild," or "free-range" on the packaging. It's an easy way to ensure that what you're buying is the best for you, your weight, and the environment.

Fiber

Fiber, the F to the P. What is required on your plate for this program? Every single meal needs to have a good-quality fiber source, just as you need a good-quality protein source. I always find it amazing that my clients are often surprised that this commonly known nutrient is such a huge component of their weight loss guidelines.

While eating fiber is certainly not a new concept, most Americans are still falling short on adequate fiber intake. This is part of the reason I was compelled to help Reserveage and their parent company Twinlab create a better fiber supplement, FibeHER (more on this on page 74). That said, this supplement is only meant to help you meet your needs every day. It is not meant to be a substitute for eating fibrous foods. The overall health benefits of fiber (which we'll talk more about in a bit) are extensive, but nothing beats fiber when it comes to weight loss and weight maintenance.

Fiber Options and Serving Sizes

You'll notice that this list doesn't include every vegetable out there. I picked the best low-sugar, high-fiber options for you, but it's OK to opt for items that aren't on the list.

Fruit

1 medium apple or pear

1 orange or tangerine

2 clementines

½ cup berries, grapes, or melon

½ grapefruit

1 peach, nectarine, or plum

Vegetables

Broccoli (unlimited)

Cauliflower (unlimited)

Spinach, kale, Swiss chard (unlimited)

Lettuce (unlimited)

Brussels sprouts (unlimited)

Asparagus (unlimited)

1 large artichoke

1 cup zucchini

1 cup eggplant

1 cup mushrooms

1 cup bell peppers

Fiber is one of the three pillars that help slow down the absorption of sugar, along with protein and fat. That's why eating a piece of fruit is so much smarter than drinking juice. Since juice has no fiber, its natural sugars—which exist even if no sugar is added—get absorbed super-quickly into your bloodstream, causing a hormonal response and sugar spike in the body, and then most often get stored as fat. Eating a piece of fruit, on the other hand, especially a high-fiber fruit, will slow down the absorption, allowing your blood sugar levels to remain more stable and setting up your body to use the sugar for energy instead of storing it as fat.

There are actually two types of fiber, soluble (nuts, seeds, beans, barley) and insoluble (spinach, kale, celery, eggplant). An ideal diet has a nice mix of the two. Both types of fiber leave you feeling fuller and more satisfied from your meal. They slow down the absorption of sugar into your bloodstream and support weight loss by helping with appetite control. In fact, many studies have shown the connection between fiber intake and a lower body weight. The theories behind this connection between fiber and lower body weight are based on satiety and blood sugar control, as well as caloric control—as many high-fiber foods are low in calories.

Not only does fiber offer weight loss benefits, but it is actually the healthiest nutrient out there. While it is certainly not sexy to talk about, insoluble fiber basically helps you poop. (Everybody poops. I am literally paid to talk about pooping—lucky me!) Insoluble fiber helps move waste through your GI system, preventing constipation, indigestion, and that unpleasant bloated feeling.

Fiber is also heart-healthy. Soluble fiber, in particular, helps lower cholesterol levels and lower your risk of high blood pressure. It can also help prevent diabetes and metabolic syndrome since it has a healthy influence on blood sugar levels. Studies have also shown that there is an inverse association between blood sugar levels and dietary fiber, which means a high-fiber diet may help prevent insulin resistance. This basically means a high-fiber diet can help prevent diabetes.

Keeping your gut filled with high-fiber foods is also a great way to keep your gut microbiome happy and healthy. You will read more about the importance of prebiotics and probiotics later, in the chapter on supplements (see "Happy Gut"

More Fiber = More H_2O

When you increase your fiber intake, you must also increase your water intake. Fiber absorbs water in your GI tract, and without sufficient water, fiber will constipate you instead of helping you poop. Aim for at least eight 8-ounce glasses a day.

on page 79), but basically a high-fiber diet is the ideal food for maintaining a thriving population of healthy bacteria. And studies show that a healthy gut is linked to a healthy weight and a strong immune system.

Fiber is found in fruits, vegetables, and whole grains. Since for this program we consider whole grains a starch (see "Rule #2: Check Your Starches" on page 40), for our purposes when we discuss fiber, we are pretty much talking about fruits and vegetables. However, it's important to note that some vegetables, like potatoes, sweet potatoes, butternut squash, and corn, also get put into the starch category due to their high carbohydrate content.

Q. I know it's good for me, but will it make me skinny?

A. I have one girlfriend who asks me this question about every new food product I discover. Her priority is losing weight and changing her appearance rather than improving her health, and I always have to explain to her that if you want to look good and be at a healthy weight, then you need to eat healthy food. Smart food choices, like having protein and fiber at every meal, are the key to achieving your ideal weight.

While I rarely allow clients to eat huge portions of anything, for the most part eating extra amounts of high-fiber vegetables is basically always OK. I would also be really impressed if I could find someone who overate broccoli, cauliflower, kale, or any other greens. (On a personal note, I can polish off an entire head of broccoli or cauliflower that's been roasted. I don't mean to brag, but it's one of my superpowers!)

Rule #1 Summary

Every meal needs to have a protein option (animal-based or plant-based) and a fiber option.

Rule #2
Check Your Starches

For the most part, this diet plan doesn't call for counting calories, points, or really almost anything except for starches. Every single one of my clients, especially my weight-loss clients, has a number of servings of starches allotted to him or her daily. During your one-week Kick-Starter program, I allotted you one starch a day. One serving of rice, quinoa, bread, wraps, or sweet potato. Pretty restrictive, right? Let's discuss why I wanted you to rein it in on the starch.

First, let's talk about what a starch is and why I call it that. The notion of a low-carb diet gets thrown around all the time. Clients come into my office and say they're on a low-carb diet, just like they say they don't eat sugar. But they're still eating things like fruits, vegetables, and dairy (fruits, veggies, and dairy are all technically carbs, and fruits and many dairy products contain sugar). So I know I need to clarify what I mean when I say "starch" and why I use this term rather than "carbs." Because my ultimate goal with this diet plan is to make all of this as simple as possible for you.

Carbohydrates are a type of macronutrient (the other two macronutrients are protein and fat). They're found in foods like fruits, vegetables, grains, and dairy products. So eating these foods does not constitute a low-carb diet. When people are avoiding breadlike products, what they're really avoiding are starchy foods. These foods include grains and all flour products, like bread, pasta, and cereal. Along with higher-carbohydrate and higher-sugar vegetables (such as corn, winter squash, peas, and potatoes), I have put these foods into the starch category to make things as simple as possible. They get looped in together because of the way the body breaks down and absorbs the nutrients they provide.

The foods that I have categorized as starches get broken down quickly and absorbed by the body as sugar. Basically, the body's goal when breaking down any of the foods we consume is to break them down into sugar so they can be used as energy or stored as fat. Since starches are easy to overeat, we tend to consume too much of them and then our body is flooded with too much sugar. As we discussed in the previous section, this triggers insulin, and the body goes into fat-storing mode.

Why are these foods so easy to overeat? The sugar content is the main reason. Since starches don't naturally contain much protein or fat, they're absorbed quickly into the bloodstream. And foods that are absorbed quickly by the bloodstream are considered to have what's called a "high glycemic index." The glycemic index is a value ranging from 0 to 100 that indicates just how much a food can spike your blood sugar. Pure sugar has a glycemic index of 100. Your average whole-wheat bread has a glycemic index of 71, while plain chicken has a glycemic index of 0. A study published in the *American Journal of Clinical Nutrition* compared a low-glycemic-index meal to an equal-calorie high-glycemic-index meal and found that the high-glycemic-index meal was associated with increased levels of hunger and cravings after the meal, which led to poor food choices at the next meal. Basically, eating a meal with a higher glycemic index literally made people hungrier and want to eat more or make worse choices at the next meal. Consider this when it comes to what time of day you eat your starches too. Another study published in *Pediatrics* concluded that high-glycemic-index meals led to a hormonal and metabolic reaction that led to excessive food intake in obese subjects. This is one of the many reasons why I recommend saving your starches for later in the day (see "Rule #3: Clock Your Meals" on page 46). Consuming your starch in the morning can trigger your appetite and prevent you from making a healthier choice at your next meal or snack. All of this is the reasoning behind my starch quota for my clients.

Even though I don't require that you give up starches completely in order to lose weight and keep it off, this is the one food category that I require tracking, because of how easy they are to overeat—and how that can affect subsequent food choices.

Aside from the fact that starch is easy to overeat, there are other reasons why I've instituted a starch quota. Many studies have shown that a diet lower in carbohydrates and low on the glycemic index is the best for weight loss and weight maintenance. I've seen the same thing in my own practice. Back in the nineties, fat was considered the main enemy. We lived on fat-free food in hopes that our waistlines would shrink and our risk of heart disease would decrease. But we were all duped, and during this time of a fat-free world, we got fatter and our hearts got sicker. As I discussed earlier in this chapter, it was sugar, not fat, that caused all this. Remember, though, that even nonsweet foods have lots of sugar in them, and that's where the starch restrictions come in.

Somehow with the low-carb craze (which isn't necessarily a bad thing in my mind), people began to have a terrible relationship with starches. What happened is that they became so forbidden that all of a sudden eating a slice of bread was considered the equivalent of eating a slice of cake. New clients come into my practice and say that they've often tried to give up bread or pasta but they've ended up overeating or even bingeing on it. When something becomes so forbidden that it causes a rebound effect, I know that the philosophy is off.

There are some diets out there that completely eliminate carbohydrates. While we certainly don't need them in our diet because we can get all the same nutrients from other foods, the problem is a behavioral one. When a stale piece of bread from the breadbasket becomes a forbidden fruit, I know this isn't working. My job is to help people create behaviors that can last for a lifetime, and excluding a huge food group isn't something that can work for everyone over a sustained period of time. Eating proper amounts of these starches can also be a very effective method of weight loss; hence the popularity of an Atkins-style diet. But when you ban an entire food group, from a behavioral standpoint you set people up to fail and rebound and yo-yo. That's not long-term weight loss or maintenance. And that's why watching your starch portions is a great way to lose weight and keep it off. Studies have compared low-fat diets (no, thank you) and low-carb diets, and numerous studies have shown that low-carbohydrate diets are more effective for weight loss and maintaining the weight loss plus reducing cardiovascular risk factors.

So how many servings of starches can you eat in a day? If you're actively trying to lose weight, your starch number would ideally be one per day when possible, and no more than two. If you're at a healthy weight already and working on maintaining it, you can eat two or sometimes three starches per day. It's not a free-for-all, though—with the portions I give you, a simple sandwich would count as two starches.

So it's really important to remember just exactly what a starch serving in the Diet Detox program looks like. And always opt for the best-quality starches you can. Avoid white-flour products when possible so you at least get some fiber and nutrients from your starch. So choose multigrain bread over white bread, whole-wheat pasta over regular white-flour pasta. In fact, all white-flour products (not white rice though!) count as intentional indulgences here (see "Rule #6: Indulge Intentionally" on page 68). Good-quality whole-grain options, on the other hand, are starches. Don't confuse the two!

If you don't agree that's it's easy to overeat starches, take a look at the serving sizes in the sidebar to the right. A serving of pasta is only ⅔ cup and most restaurants serve a portion that is three times that amount. Or consider the fact that a typical bagel is actually equivalent to five slices of bread. So while there is still a place for your favorite starches (see "Step Rule #6: Indulge Intentionally" on page 68), a starch that's portioned out correctly may look different than what you're used to eating.

I am often asked about giving up grains or gluten for health reasons. As I said earlier in this section, they're actually not necessary for our bodies to survive. Some research has indicated that giving up grains and gluten can reduce inflammation, improve brain health, and much more. Whenever I have a client who is struggling with an autoimmune illness or having inexplicable symptoms, after making sure the rest of his or her diet is on point, I'll often take away grains and/or dairy to see if there is any improvement within a month. If people see

Starch Options and Serving Sizes

1 slice of multigrain bread*

½ cup (cooked) rice (white, brown, or black)

1 tortilla/wrap*

1 small or ½ large sweet potato, potato

⅔ cup (cooked) pasta*

½ cup (cooked) oatmeal

1 roll or 4 pieces sushi

½ cup winter squash

½ cup or 1 small ear corn

½ cup peas

2 cups popcorn

½ cup beans**

*See brands I love on page 197.

**Beans are a tricky situation—they're high in carbohydrates but also contain a nice amount of protein and fiber. My rule: If beans are your only protein source, then they count as your protein for that meal. If there is another protein option (think turkey chili), then they count as your starch for that meal.

Case Study: Alison

My first session with Alison was pretty typical—when I asked her about her current eating habits, Alison told me that in order to lose weight she doesn't touch bread or pasta or "any of that good stuff." I should add that Alison was also more than 50 pounds overweight. So I pressed her, asking about how she got to her current weight. She told me that she loses her willpower and starts to eat "all the carbs." This is a typical example of what I see in my practice regularly. Alison had determined that the only way she could lose weight was by summoning up a ton of willpower and avoiding "all the carbs" until she lost weight.

As a serial dieter, Alison wasn't impressed by my first few rules. I knew she was skeptical and wanted me to be stricter and give her some insane plan to follow. Furthermore, she didn't understand how I could let her eat a starch, not to mention two starches, every day—and still expect the scale to move. I asked her to trust me and to come back the next week.

When Alison came back the following week, we had a good session. She said that the rules had seemed so simple at first, but that when she put them into action, she realized the program was a bigger overhaul than she had expected (happens every time!). More important, she said that in the first few days she was both excited and nervous about eating her starches; she was concerned that the scale wouldn't go down, or at least wouldn't move as quickly as it would if she were still eating some of these "carby" foods. When I weighed her after just one week, she had lost 4 pounds! This was when I knew that I could finally rid this woman of the notion that she needed to depend on willpower instead of making smart decisions. After a few weeks on this plan, Alison was already down 20 pounds. When she came in for her fifth session, she told me that the starches (she was finally not calling them "carbs") had lost a lot of their allure. Because she was eating sweet potatoes, rice, quinoa, and good-quality bread, starches had become just another element on her plate rather than something special. Her cravings for them and her behavior toward them had changed simply because we had taken them off the pedestal. Because she made healthy starch options a regular part of her eating, the unhealthy starches that she used to binge on were no longer as appealing. It turned out that Alison didn't need more willpower—she just needed to stop dieting. After six months with me Alison was down 53 pounds, and she has now maintained this loss for almost two years.

improvements from a grain-free and gluten-free diet, I keep them off those foods. Most people feel better overall when they begin to watch their portions and the quality of their grain and starch choices. Plain old white flour is incredibly inflammatory and provides your body with very little nutritional value. My only concern, as I've mentioned numerous times, is the behavioral side of this all. I would much rather have a client who eats small portions of good-quality starches regularly than one who tries to avoid starches but then has a showdown with a bowl of pasta. The best part of not being so crazy restrictive with my clients is that this freedom gives them a better source of control plus takes a lot of these foods off the pedestal that they've been put on.

Q. Are gluten-free pretzels, crackers, and other snacks a better option?

A. Organic, gluten-free, Paleo, vegan—all these terms come with a "health halo," meaning people automatically assume they are healthy. Gluten-free pretzels or organic pretzels are still just a carby/starchy snack that does nothing for you nutrition-wise. I would much rather you snack on carrots and hummus. Do not let flashy labels fool you into thinking you are eating something healthier than it is. If you would not eat it without the special label, then do not eat it at all.

 Rule #2 Summary

Have no more than two servings of starch a day, and make sure they are good-quality, whole-grain options or starchy vegetables.

Rule #3
Clock Your Meals

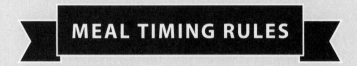

MEAL TIMING RULES

1. Eat a meal or a snack every 4 hours.
2. Make breakfast substantial and starch-free.
3. Leave at least 12 to 14 hours between your dinner and the following breakfast.

The ultimate goal of any diet plan that will lead to long-term success is to keep your blood sugar as stable as possible. Nothing good happens when your blood sugar is on a roller coaster of highs and lows, and unpleasant feelings are created, as aptly described by my favorite word, *hangry*. That's the main reasoning behind this rule. Each meal or snack is the opportunity to set yourself up for success. By enjoying a satisfying breakfast, eating consistently, and giving yourself time to digest overnight, you will be doing just that. Having a meal or a snack about every 4 hours allows your body to be fueled without creating the urge to overeat, which is what happens when you allow too much time to pass between meals.

My clients joke that they are always eating on my plan, and while, yes, there is no meal skipping allowed and I do want you to eat some snacks, I want to make it very clear that there is a firm difference between eating regularly and grazing all day. It's important that there is a start and an end to every meal and snack.

Case Study: Tom

Tom is a client who has a pretty hectic work schedule and a fast-paced job. He travels a lot, and when he's at his office he's swamped. When I first met Tom, he was having a decent breakfast at his desk around 7:00 AM. It was often eggs, toast, and maybe a smoothie. Then that was it for the rest of the day. Around 3:00 or 4:00 PM he'd break open his desk stash of candy and eat that to power through the rest of the day. He wouldn't have another structured meal until a late dinner after he left the office. Tom was only about 15 pounds overweight, but he felt terrible. He had bags under his eyes and wasn't sleeping well. Going over his food journal, I saw red flags popping up everywhere. I'm sure even as a reader you already see the major holes in his diet. Tom did not. Tom had convinced himself that it was better to keep working through his meals instead of taking a few minutes for a break to actually eat some food. As a result, he felt and looked terrible.

Snacking

Snacks don't have to include both a protein and a fiber source. One or the other is good enough as long as your meals contain both.

I knew Tom would be all about efficiency, so I had to come up with a plan that would be easy for him to follow. The first step was to get him to eat a meal or a snack every 4 hours. Then we came up with easy meal ideas. Since Tom picked up his breakfast on his way to work, that was the time to also pick up his lunch and/or snacks for the day. He could get a wrap or a salad and not have to think about lunch once it was time, because the food was already there. He could even buy nuts, yogurt, or jerky in the morning too so he was stocked for snacks. I gave him my suggestions for the best kinds of snack bars and told them they should be replacing his afternoon candy stash. These were all basic moves that would set him up for a successful day of eating but that wouldn't require any extra time aside from a few minutes in the morning. We worked on some of his other issues as well, like sleeping, hydrating, and getting to the gym, but the major change for Tom involved eating in between breakfast and dinner.

Within one month, Tom had lost almost 10 pounds and was feeling better than ever. Because his blood sugar levels were staying more consistent throughout the day, he was able to focus better at work—a bonus, as he wasn't even aware that his concentration had been impaired. By taking just a few extra minutes in the morning, Tom was able to give himself more hours in his day to accomplish what he needed to do. Two months after our initial consultation, Tom had lost 18 pounds and was in better shape than ever. He said he now had the energy to go to the gym more frequently and felt better than he had in years.

Grazing Versus the 4-Hour Rule

Grazing Day

7:30 AM: Scrambled eggs with salsa

9:00 AM: Banana and a handful of almonds

11:00 AM: Apple and more almonds

2:00 PM: Half a turkey sandwich

3:30 PM: 1 tablespoon of almond butter

4:45 PM: Cookie

7:30 PM: Grilled chicken over brown rice with sautéed broccoli and cauliflower

This grazing day is filled with mainly healthy foods, yet the day consisted of nonstop eating. Sometimes it's less about the food choices and more about the details of how we're eating. Grazing can prevent us from being fully in touch with our hunger levels, which can lead to overeating. When you're constantly eating, you never actually get hungry, which means you never have to make smart, intentional decisions about your food. I bet that if the client who recorded the grazing day ate a bigger breakfast with the addition of fiber—for example, she could have sautéed veggies with her eggs and salsa—then she would be able to wait until later in the morning for her first snack, instead of needing two morning snacks. I'd also likely recommend that she (if possible) push back her lunchtime to noon to help make each meal more finite and get out of the grazing pattern.

Good Day

7:30 AM: Two-egg omelet with spinach, topped with sliced avocado

12:00 PM: Grilled chicken over salad with cucumber, tomato, feta, onion, olive oil, lemon, and salt and 10 Mary's Gone Crackers

3:15 PM: Hummus and carrots

6:30 PM: Poached salmon over steamed spinach and quinoa

Here, there's a really nice balance of protein and fiber at each meal, even in the snacks, which helped lead to smart decisions and finite meals. And I love the squeezed-in snack in the morning, since lunch was going to be on the later side.

The best way to set yourself up for success at each meal or snack is to not let yourself get so hungry that you can't make a good decision. Nothing ruins a meal like getting to the table and eating the contents of the breadbasket first thing. Reminder: The breadbasket is hardly ever worth it—don't fool yourself! The most effective way of doing this is to eat relatively frequently, approximately every 4 hours. Do you need to set an alarm and eat every 4 hours on the dot? No. You'll see in the "Good Day" above that it's not exactly every 4 hours (though it's pretty close). But some awareness is important here. If breakfast is around 7:00 am for you and lunch isn't until 1:00 pm, then it's necessary to have a snack in between. You can't make it through the morning, thinking on your feet and managing until lunch, unless you've given your body some fuel to make it through that time. I would certainly say 6 hours is too long in between meals at this time of day. However, if you eat a large breakfast (yes, please) at 7:00 am and then eat lunch at noon, you can go that long without a snack as long as you don't feel too hungry before lunch.

Favorite Bars

While I'd much prefer that everyone had healthy, whole-food snacks handy in the afternoon, it's not always possible. That's when a snack bar is super-helpful. But some of these bars can be so high in sugar that you might as well be eating a candy bar. Here are some of my favorite bars, which should be kept in your office drawer, your gym bag, or your purse. Some do have sugar, but because it's so balanced with protein, fiber, or fat, I'm OK with these options. Plus, you can find these in pretty much any grocery store (and some gas stations).

Elemental Superfood Seedbar, Health Warrior Chia Bar, Kind, Lärabar, Perfect Bar, Raw Crunch, Wild Zora

The midafternoon snack is crucial here. Around 3:00 or 4:00 pm is a hard time for many people, and nothing good happens if you're not set up for success. You'll know who isn't prepared by seeing which of your colleagues sneak off to the vending machine, indulge in the office cupcakes, or grab another cup of coffee and throw in a cookie at the last minute. It's because their blood sugar is dropping, and we don't make smart decisions when our blood sugar isn't stable.

> *"The Diet Detox has been my driving force for feeling healthy. The balanced meals and simple rules helped me say goodbye to my years of yo-yo dieting. I never realized how strong the correlation between eating healthy and feeling healthy really is until the Diet Detox."*
>
> —Tracy L., sales manager

Making Breakfast Substantial—Ideally Without Starch

There's an old saying that goes, "Eat breakfast like a king, lunch like a prince, and dinner like a pauper." While I don't think that dinner needs to be super-tiny, I agree that breakfast needs to be substantial. Numerous studies have shown the benefits of a larger, healthy breakfast. One study published in the *International Journal of Obesity* showed that when subjects were given the same exact meal for breakfast or dinner, the people receiving the meal for breakfast had better metabolic reactions than those eating the meal for dinner. They were eating the same exact meal, but the difference was the timing. We want our metabolism to work in our favor, and having a large breakfast is a great way to get it going in the right direction. Another study showed that eating a big "high-energy" breakfast and a smaller dinner can help control blood sugar levels in obese nondiabetic individuals. Blood sugar stabilization is the key in any healthy meal plan. So what does a big breakfast look like? It's certainly not a stack of pancakes. It's a meal with a protein and a fiber on your plate or in your bowl. Don't overthink it—just eat it.

Here are some examples:

Breakfast protein options: eggs, nuts, nut butter, full-fat yogurt, turkey, cheese, smoked salmon, chia seeds

Breakfast fiber options: fruit, nonstarchy vegetables, chia seeds

Fruit is a great fiber option in the morning and most people enjoy it with breakfast. I don't restrict which types of fruit you can eat too much, but it's wise to opt for the lower-sugar fruits whenever possible, especially in the morning. While I'd rather you ate a banana than a bagel in the morning, I'd still prefer an apple or berries (my favorite low-sugar fruits) over

Cereal Alternatives

These must be eaten with a protein source!

Nature's Path Qi'a, Purely Elizabeth Ancient Grain Granola, WholeMe Clusters

the banana due to the banana's higher sugar content and higher glycemic index. A study published in 2017 in the *American Journal of Clinical Nutrition* linked higher-sugar fruit to a higher risk of diabetes. When in doubt, always opt for fruit over another option, but if you can have your pick of the bunch, aim for the lower-sugar fruits whenever possible, especially in the morning.

One thing you won't see here is cold cereal. Aside from obviously being a starch, most cold cereal is loaded with sugar (even the ones without marshmallows), low in protein, and lacking in significant fiber. Cereal is one of those meals that you eat and then shortly afterwards feel hungry again. When you are further along in the Diet Detox—after you have lost some weight and gotten the hang of the rules—then maybe you can consider adding a cereal as one of your intentional indulgences. Alternatively, there are a few healthy granola-style cereals out there that are great for sprinkling on top of yogurt for a snack; this cereal and yogurt combo is my only exception to the no-cereal rule, simply because of the nutritional profile of good-quality protein, fiber, and fat—and the fact that it is super-yummy!

Getting Dinner Right

I'm just going to be blunt here: big dinners eaten late in the evening do nothing for you or your waistline. Eating a large meal before you go to bed can lead to everything from heartburn and acid reflux to weight gain. Because your body isn't usually active post-dinner, the food you eat isn't used for energy, so it automatically heads to fat storage. Think about that study in the *International Journal of Obesity* I mentioned earlier: the same meal, when eaten for dinner instead of breakfast, had a different effect on the participants' metabolism, resulting in a slower caloric burn. Dinner is still important, but it shouldn't be a giant, heavy meal.

Often my clients are too tired by the time they get home at the end of the day to want to think about dinner. Luckily the protein and fiber tool makes it easy to do the right thing. Piece of chicken? Check. Some frozen spinach to defrost? Check. Some leftover quinoa? Check. The meal is done. It doesn't need to be overthought. Make sure that each category of protein, fiber, and (if you have not already eaten your two-serving daily maximum) starch is checked and move on. Try to save your starches for dinner whenever possible. It sets you up for a better night's sleep because the carbohydrates can help you fall asleep more quickly, plus it's a nice way to end the day.

Then there's the issue of how late you're eating. Part of the "clock your meals" rule is the principle of leaving a minimum of 12 to 14 hours between dinner and the following breakfast. This is because of one diet trend that I haven't spoken about yet that the science nerd in me thinks is pretty cool: intermittent fasting. Fasting is defined as not having any food for a period of time, whether it's two days a week or 16 hours between meals. The science behind the benefits of intermittent fasting is solid, and evidence points toward benefits such as weight loss, reduced risk of type 2 diabetes, and improved heart health. While that's all very compelling, it's hard and restrictive, and I find that when a program is that restrictive, it often sets you up to fail. Yet I can't look past the science, so I figured out a way to incorporate some of the benefits of intermittent fasting into a sustainable diet program (hello, Diet Detox). That's the theory behind eating an earlier dinner and aiming to get close to 12 to 14 hours between dinner and breakfast. A study published in *Cell Metabolism* showed that regardless of what diet plan mice were put on, mice that were given restricted time windows of 9, 10, and 12 hours to eat (i.e., only eating between 7:00 AM and 4:00 PM or 7:00 AM and 7:00 PM) developed less body fat than mice that ate all day long, even though they all ate the same number of calories.

Another version of intermittent fasting is called early time-restricted feeding (eTRF), and it's a similar concept to my 12- to 14-hour rule. eTRF is a bit stricter as it prescribes that you eat your last meal in the midafternoon and then not eat again until the next morning. The findings on this concept were presented at the Obesity Society Annual Meeting in the fall of 2016 by a team of researchers from Pennington Biomedical Research

Center, who concluded that eating for a small window of time, approximately 8:00 AM to 2:00 PM, can greatly help with weight loss by optimizing metabolic functions; this is partially because food is consumed at the time of day when the body's metabolism is most efficient.

But we're not mice, and fasting all day or skipping dinner isn't going to work for the majority of us. However, the science is pretty cool and solid. That's where my expertise comes in. My strong suit is helping my clients figure out what works best for them specifically and how to keep at it. If people won't be able to realistically stick to a program, or if a program causes them to make poor food choices as a rebound effect, then it doesn't matter how good the science is. So how do you take this info

Let's Get Personal

Everyone who knows me well knows that I don't do evenings. I don't eat late—I don't eat dinner out past 7:00 PM—and I don't stay up late. It's a bit challenging socially, but I get to have fun with friends and then, shamelessly, I am always the first to leave. I own it, they get it, and it's not a big deal. Join me in transforming the early-bird special into something that is not just for seniors! If you have to eat a late dinner, eat breakfast later to give yourself that extra time and then skip your midmorning snack.

and make it work for you? It's the 12- to 14-hour window. By taking a 12- to 14-hour break between dinner and breakfast, you get not only the metabolic boost of an earlier dinner but also some of the same benefits you would get from hard-core intermittent fasting or from eTRF, although without any of the hunger pains or rebound-bingeing side effects.

I like to give my clients a "kitchen curfew." This is primarily for those who tend to stay up later, as those evening hours are when they start creeping back into the kitchen. So give yourself a kitchen curfew. Shut it down after your early dinner. Tea or water is OK, but floss and brush your teeth early to prevent those extra unnecessary snacks, so you can give your body those 12 to 14 hours as a break between meals. On top of that, I'm asking you to have your last meal of the day on the earlier side whenever possible. Remember, I'm a realist; I understand that not everyone can be done eating by 7:00 PM, but whenever possible, aim for it. Then give your body at least 90 minutes to 2 hours from when you ate until you go to sleep.

This rule isn't hard to follow. All I'm asking you here in this "Clock Your Meals" section is to eat a big breakfast, snack every 4 hours, and have dinner on the earlier side. That's all it takes to see some major benefits. Add this one to all the other changes you're making and results will happen even quicker!

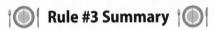 **Rule #3 Summary**

Eat a meal or a snack approximately every 4 hours. Make breakfast substantial and starch-free, and leave at least 12 to 14 hours between your dinner and the following breakfast.

Rule #4
Eat Fat

I say this again and again in my office, during media interviews, and to anyone who asks: fat does not make you fat. In fact, fat can do just the opposite. Fat is so important to have in our daily diets: it makes food taste better, and it's satisfying and satiating. When clients come to me after years of eating low-fat or fat-free foods, I feel like I'm breaking them out of their fat-free prisons. Fat-free cookies, skim milk, and fat-free salad dressing are all just plain old nonsense.

Where did this fat phobia come from? Turns out it was all a scam starting way back in the 1950s. Some scientists manipulated data to make a connection between fat and heart disease. In fact, there's evidence that some sugar industry honchos were actually paying scientists to alter their data and to blame fat for the problems in the world, specifically the obesity epidemic and the rise of heart disease. Thus began years of fat-free living. Guess what happened to obesity and heart disease rates? They didn't go down; they went *up*. In order to make food products palatable and give them a shelf life when fat was removed, manufacturers replaced it with sugar. As you'll see in the section on Rule #5, sugar, not fat, is the underlying cause of obesity and heart disease. I have memories of my grandfather eating his All-Bran cereal with water because he was so scared of fat and its effect on heart disease. Did you know that the second ingredient in All-Bran is sugar? It would have been better for him to eat eggs—yolks and all—than cereal with water.

Aside from weight gain, everyone's fear of fat stems from its connection to heart disease. Numerous studies, many of them meta-analyses of cohort studies that are the gold standard of scientific literature, show there is no significant evidence that dietary saturated fat is linked to heart disease. Several other studies even suggest that saturated fats can actually *reduce* the risk of suffering a stroke. The only fats that I strongly recommend you avoid are trans-fatty acids, which come from processed vegetable oils.

Healthy Sources of Fat

Avocado, grass-fed butter, olive oil, ghee, coconut oil, eggs, grass-fed beef

You'll mainly see them listed on labels as "partially hydrogenated oil," and they can be found in processed baked goods, fried foods, and some nondairy creamers or butter substitutes. Trans-fatty acids can increase your risk of heart disease—these are the fats you should stay away from!

How does a diet rich in saturated fats help your body? The ultimate goal of a healthy diet is for your food to be digested slowly, so that the sugar you consume is in turn absorbed slowly. That allows your blood sugar levels to remain steady and your body to utilize insulin properly. Fat has a great impact on insulin levels, allowing them to remain on the lower side, which keeps diabetes at bay. This is because fat slows down the absorption of sugar in the body.

Also, since fat is much more satiating, you're more likely to eat less of your food when fat is involved. Studies have even shown that when fat replaces sugar in the diet, people tend to eat less, which has a positive influence on their weight. Eating fat actually has a direct effect on your appetite. It triggers the release of a hormone called cholecystokinin, which causes the feeling of fullness. Fat is also important to have in your meals to help you properly absorb all the nutrients in your food. Certain vitamins are considered fat-soluble vitamins because they can only be absorbed into the body when consumed with fat—specifically vitamins A, D, E, and K. These vitamins are required for your body to function effectively, and they provide your body with some major health benefits. They are necessary for antioxidant utilization, hormonal regulation, bone maintenance, immune system support, and heart health.

In the diet plan, I don't have a specific requirement for how much fat you should eat. This is for two reasons: The first is that I don't want this program to be any more complicated than it needs to be. The second is that fat is not always the main ingredient—it's a vehicle to cook foods in, a dressing for a salad, or an element that adds richness to something else, like full-fat yogurt. I want you to make sure fat is part of each meal, but I don't want you to overthink it—just keep the amounts close to the recommended portion sizes. Simply cooking your vegetables in a tablespoon of coconut oil is a great way to

Coconut Water

Don't be confused by coconut water and the benefits of coconut fat. Coconut water doesn't contain any fat. But it can be a great sports drink. Just make sure to buy a version that is pure coconut water and is not mixed with other juices, which are too high in sugar.

make sure fat is in your dinner. Yes, I said coconut oil. Coconuts really got a bad rap along with eggs during the fat-free craze. They're high in saturated fat, and that seems to throw a lot of people off, but not all saturated fats are bad. Coconut—not a chocolate-covered coconut candy bar, but real coconut oil or coconut meat—is filled with medium-chain fatty acids (MCFAs). These MCFAs are smaller than other fats, are easily digested, and can even be used as energy in the body. Studies have shown that MCFAs can't be stored as fat in the body and can even promote a reduction in belly fat. Belly fat is the type of fat we all want to avoid as much as possible because it surrounds our major organs and is linked to everything from metabolic syndrome to heart disease. Another study from 2009 showed that a diet rich in coconut oil actually protects against insulin resistance and prevents extra body fat from developing. Since coconut oil has a high smoking point, it makes a great cooking oil. It doesn't have a coconutty flavor once it's cooked and is perfect for many different recipes.

"The Diet Detox is a fantastic program! Within six months I went from a size 12 to a size 6–8. People ask me all the time, 'How did you do it?' The answer is simple: the Diet Detox. The Diet Detox is not a diet but a whole new way of looking at food and learning what to eat. The Diet Detox leaves the choices up to me, giving me full control, which has been a huge part of my success."

—W. Smith, writer

Avocados are another one of my favorite fat options. You can easily throw them into a salad or a smoothie, or you can just eat them on the side for a great fat boost. A cool study from the *Nutrition Journal* came out a few years ago with evidence that adding half a Hass avocado to your lunch can help keep you fuller for the next 3 to 5 hours. Another study using eggs instead of avocados had a similar result too.

There's one other fat that I want to mention and it's chocolate. Yes, you read that right! Delicious chocolate. I'm a chocolate girl—always have been and always will be—so it wouldn't be possible for me to create a diet plan that excluded chocolate. I've even tried writing an all-chocolate diet book, but that was overboard even for me. So that's why I always allow chocolate in my programs. But let's get a few things straight here first. I'm not talking about milk chocolate or white chocolate (that's not even actual chocolate!). I'm talking about high-quality dark chocolate

Double-Duty Foods

These are protein options that also meet your fat needs.

Full-fat yogurt, eggs, nuts, nut butter, grass-fed meat, seeds, chia seeds

that is 70 percent cocoa or more. Ideally your chocolate is closer to 85 percent cocoa to help prevent overeating. Food scientists use the term *hyperpalatable* to describe a food that is easy to overeat. Chocolate with 65 percent cocoa and lower falls into the highly hyperpalatable category. Opting for dark chocolate that is 70 percent cocoa or higher allows you to enjoy the pleasures of chocolate without giving your body a sugar rush that would cause overeating. Not only is good-quality chocolate delicious, but studies have also shown that it has tons of health benefits. There's an association between chocolate consumption and a lower body weight plus a lower risk of cardiovascular disease. This positive benefit occurs because dark chocolate is loaded with antioxidants and polyphenols, which have been linked to metabolic health and heart health.

I have found that when I give clients chocolate regularly, I can get them to consistently eat properly. One client, Dina, had been on tons of diets when she first came to see me. She wouldn't even use olive oil on her salads because it would make them fattening. I had to first calm her fears of fat, and as we added it to her diet (goodbye, egg whites!) and her weight continued to go down, we made some progress. Before coming to me, Dina had never been able to stick to a diet plan. She'd lose weight for a brief period and then find her diet too restrictive and start eating all the things she missed until she was right back where she started. I knew she was a chocolate girl like me, and I told her to eat 1 ounce of dark chocolate every single day. In fact, I made her eat a piece while she was in my office, as I have a stash here at all times. When I saw her the next week, she had lost 3 more pounds and couldn't believe that she was eating chocolate every day *and* losing weight. The chocolate was enough of a treat for her (and not considered an intentional indulgence; see "Rule #6: Indulge Intentionally" on page 68) to keep her motivated to make a healthy choice at the next meal. So go ahead and

My Favorite Chocolates

Eating Evolved, Green & Black's, Hu Kitchen, Nib Mor, Sweetriot

enjoy your piece of chocolate if you like. By the way, Dina is down over 50 pounds and eats chocolate every day. Whether it's eggs, avocados, olive oil, coconut oil, or another option, fat does not make you fat.

 Rule #4 Summary

Eat at least one serving of fat with your meals. Cook your vegetables in coconut oil, use olive oil on top of your salad, or opt for full-fat dairy products.

Rule #5
Watch the Sugar

I'm basically known in my industry as the anti-sugar nutritionist. It's not the most glamorous title, but it's true. I even wrote a book against sugar called *The Sugar Detox*.

The research that I did for that book flipped everything I had learned in graduate school—and how I was raised—on its head. Sugar, not fat, was the cause of so many health problems. So was saturated fat not the bad guy anymore? Everything seemed to make sense as I put that book together. My goal was to help people with a true sugar addiction—sugar is basically just as addicting as cocaine. The research changed the way I looked at sugar, it changed the way I worked with clients, and it changed the way my family ate. I originally wanted to name that book *Sugar Makes You Fat and Old*, but I guess it didn't have that ring to it.

The first thing to clarify is that when I talk about sugar, I am mainly discussing added sugars. All too often, a client says, "I don't eat any sugar," but when I review his or her typical diet, I see it's loaded with foods like yogurt, fruit, grains, and vegetables. Natural sugars are almost everywhere, even in foods that can be good for us. They are found in all dairy products, fruits, many vegetables, and grains. For the most part, it's OK to eat these foods, providing you're following the rules of protein plus fiber plus fat throughout your day, since those three things slow down the absorption of sugar into your bloodstream.

Let's get a little scientific here for a moment. When we consume sugar, it gets digested and taken up by our bloodstream. As soon as sugar reaches our bloodstream, a hormone called insulin becomes active—this is a good thing at first. Insulin is in charge of regulating the metabolism of sugar, and its main job is to tell that sugar where to go. In an ideal setting, we consume a healthy source of sugar (a piece of fruit) and insulin says, "Hooray—let's use this for energy!" Unfortunately, when we eat large amounts of sugar frequently, we build up a surplus in our body and have more than we need

Sneaky Sources of Sugar

Snack bars, crackers, bread, barbecue sauce, ketchup, salad dressings, tomato sauce, nut butter, bottled teas, prepared smoothies, yogurt, milk chocolate, granola

Case Study: Kim

Kim was a client of mine whom I had been seeing for about six months; she had arrived around the same time that I began my research on sugar. She had been successful, losing around 15 pounds during that time, but still had another 30 pounds to go. Kim had been patient but was definitely ready for the weight to start coming off a bit more quickly. At first glance, her food diaries were solid. No major red flags at all. But the more I was reading about sugar, the more I started to realize that I was missing something in my practice, especially with Kim. Kim was eating smart portions of traditional starches, like grains. There weren't too many desserts at all, as she was happy eating fruit instead. Her only nonapproved item was a diet soda that she was drinking daily. At the time, I was picking my battles with her. Since she was able to give up dessert, I didn't want to fight the diet soda. But after everything I had been reading about sugar, it seemed to be wrong to let this keep going.

During my next appointment with Kim, I laid down the new groundwork for her. The first thing I told her was that she had to give up the diet soda. I explained that, although the diet soda might seem to be satisfying her sweet tooth in a relatively healthy or low-calorie way, it was only encouraging her sweet tooth. Artificial sweeteners aren't the answer, as they cause the same problems, if not worse ones, as regular sugar does. She laughed and asked what eating habits the diet soda could be encouraging, since she doesn't eat any sweets. That's when I started talking about her fruit intake. She ate fruit at breakfast, during her snacks, and as a dessert replacement. I gave her some new rules, all targeting the amount of sugar she was consuming, even from fruit. Plus, the diet soda was no longer allowed. When I saw her the next week, she told me she was shocked at how hard the week had been for her. She had had a headache for a few days and had been irritable with pretty much everyone, including me during that session. She was actually having slight withdrawal symptoms from sugar and artificial sweeteners. What made her less irritable was getting on the scale and seeing she had dropped 4 pounds in one week. That was double what she had been able to lose during her best weeks. After that session, we slowly reintroduced fruit in small portions, focusing on the lower-sugar options, like apples. Over the next two months, Kim lost 17 pounds. That's about the same amount that she lost in the six months before we focused on her sugar intake. Kim has gotten to her goal weight and still checks in with me once or twice a year. She has maintained her weight loss for over four years and is healthier than ever.

for energy. So that extra sugar gets told by the constantly present insulin to go hang out and wait. This is when it gets stored as fat as a reserve for the day when we might not have the abundance of food that we do now. It gets stored in our stomach, hips, thighs, butt, jowls—the works. The problem is that when insulin is active, our body goes into fat-storing mode, packing away sugar for a rainy or hungry day. In order to lose weight, we need insulin to be active for smaller periods of time. It will go back to its "resting" state when the sugar in our bloodstream is processed by our body, which is when we can go back to burning fat.

That's one of the main reasons the whole calorie concept doesn't work. You'll notice that we don't count calories at all in this plan, and I don't think you ever should. We don't eat numbers; we eat food. And if you eat a diet of 1,500 calories but it's loaded with sugar, well, guess what? You'll still gain weight. The quality of what you're eating is much more important than a calorie could ever be! The average person is eating close to 32 teaspoons of added sugar each day—that's a huge amount. The USDA recommends no more than 10 teaspoons a day, and that's still too much. All that extra sugar is doing more than just adding pounds on the scale too. It's also damaging our hearts. Once we have stored enough sugar, the liver starts to turn excess sugar into triglycerides that spill into the bloodstream and are connected to clogged arteries and an increased risk of heart attack. The Nurses Health Study, with over a quarter million participants, is one of the largest studies of risk factors for major chronic diseases in women. Information from this study, published in the *American Journal of Clinical Nutrition*, showed that women who ate a diet higher in sugar than that of other women had double the risk of heart disease. Let me rephrase that—a diet high in sugar is directly linked to an increased risk for heart disease. Not saturated fat, not regular fat, but sugar.

Oh, there's more too! When we eat a lot of sugar and insulin is constantly being activated in the bloodstream by our sugar intake, insulin becomes less effective. It's like when I'm yelling at my kids all day—they just hear me less and less. The yelling is no longer effective. Same deal with insulin. The more it's yelling at the sugar and telling it where to go, the less the sugar listens. That's when we become insulin resistant. The body becomes basically deaf to insulin, and this causes more sugar to run rampant in the bloodstream. The body is still desperately releasing insulin, hoping the sugar will finally listen, but it doesn't. So a vicious cycle develops in which the body stays in fat-storing mode, leading to serious health conditions such as metabolic syndrome. Metabolic syndrome is a precursor to type 2 diabetes and heart disease and now affects over 34 percent of Americans, according to the National Health and Nutrition Examination Survey (NHANES).

I think I've made myself pretty clear: sugar isn't good for you. But why is it so hard to quit? It's because the body reacts to sugar as though it were a drug. A study published in *Neuroscience & Biobehavioral Reviews* showed that sugar cravings were as demanding if not more demanding than cocaine cravings. When we eat sugar, it targets our brain by releasing opioids and dopamine, which both trigger those feel-good emotions. Sugar literally makes us feel better when we eat it by stimulating the brain's pleasure center. But that happy feeling doesn't last, so we start to crash, leading us to want more sugar, creating a vicious cycle.

Here are my three very basic rules for reducing the amount of sugar in your diet. As I've said before, there is always a place for a piece of cake; it's just not meant to be eaten every day. By following these rules, not only will you be eating less sugar, but you'll have room for these indulgences when they're worth it.

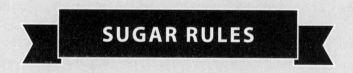

SUGAR RULES

1. Stop *adding* sugar.
2. Opt for "plain" or "unsweetened."
3. Always read the ingredients.

Sugar isn't always easy to spot. I mentioned added sugars earlier and I want to elaborate more on that. When I refer to added sugars, I'm talking about a few things: the sugar you add to your coffee, the sugar you pour on top of your oatmeal, and the sugar that you don't even know you're eating.

But First, Coffee

I always recommend iced coffee at first when nixing the sugar—unsweetened iced coffee is much more palatable than unsweetened hot coffee. And remember that it's OK to have whole milk in it too!

So my first rule when it comes to sugar is to stop *adding* sugar to your diet when it's not necessary. In coffee especially! It's not supposed to be a coffee-flavored milk shake! My head spins when I see someone walking out of Starbucks with a coffee drink covered in whipped cream. Just because it's coffee doesn't make it OK! Drink coffee with milk or cream if you want (remember, fat is OK; see "Rule #4: Eat Fat" on page 55), but for the love of all things healthy, stop adding sugar to your coffee. This includes artificial sweeteners as well; I'll go into that more in a moment. If most Americans would just stop adding sweeteners to their coffee, I bet the average weight in the United States would go down in a month.

My second rule is to think about the times you add sugar to other foods. Are you making healthy oatmeal unhealthy by pouring maple syrup all over it?

My third rule: Always read the ingredient label (not the nutrition label!). Take a look at the foods in your fridge and pantry that come in a package. Yogurt, pasta sauce, salad dressing, even bread—all these items can have added sugars in them. Check the ingredient list for words that sound like sugar. Even healthy-sounding things like "brown rice syrup" are codes for sugar. And organic sugar is still sugar regardless of whether it's organic, so don't fool yourself that it's any healthier!

If you're following the rules and reading the ingredients, your life will be slightly less sweet but a whole lot healthier (which is pretty sweet in and of itself). I prefer to always focus on the foods you should be eating regularly rather than the foods you should omit, so you feel less deprived, but there are a few items that need to be discussed and are nonnegotiable (don't even use them for an intentional indulgence): soda and artificial sweeteners.

I make a deal with all my clients that if they want to continue to be patients in my practice, they have to give up all soda and artificial sweeteners. In all honesty, I feel like I shouldn't even have to write this section because everyone should know this, but since I get asked about it all the time, here's the deal.

Regular soda has no nutritional purpose other than to get sugar into your bloodstream as quickly as possibly. It does absolutely nothing positive for your body, and the chemicals that it contains are legitimately harmful. No soda. I had a client ask me about organic soda and I laughed and laughed. Yes, it's better to have organic cane sugar than high-fructose corn syrup, but it's still sugar, and it still goes directly into your bloodstream. So just no. That said, flavored sparkling waters—so long as they don't contain sweeteners of any kind, real or artificial—are fine by me. I personally love having a stash in the fridge.

And what about artificial sweeteners? All those pretty, colorful packets that are everywhere are terrible for you. Some are believed to cause cancer, while others have been shown to alter your microbiome, or the population of friendly bacteria in your gut. Anything that messes with your microbiome is something you need to stay away from because that's the hub of not only your digestive health but also your immune system and neurological function. A study that will be presented by a team from George Washington University at ENDO 2017, the Endocrine Society's 99th annual meeting, states that there is scientific evidence that artificial sweeteners promote metabolic dysfunction, which basically causes the body to make more fat. No, thank you! As if that weren't enough, according to the *Journal of General Internal Medicine*, the Women's Health Initiative Observational Study, one of the most comprehensive studies with almost 60,000 women participating over nine years, found that participants who drank two or more cans of diet soda

Different Names for Sugar

Common Names for Sugar

Anhydrous dextrose, brown sugar, cane sugar, corn sweetener, corn syrup, corn syrup solids, crystal dextrose, crystals, evaporated cane juice, fructose sweetener, fruit juice concentrates, high-fructose corn syrup, honey, lactose, liquid fructose, malt syrup, maltose, maple syrup, molasses, pancake syrup, raw sugar, sugar, syrup, white sugar

Less Common Names for Sugar

Carbitol, concentrated fruit juice, corn sweetener, diglycerides, disaccharides, evaporated cane juice, erythritol, Florida Crystals, fructooligosaccharides, galactose, glucitol, glucosamine, hexitol, inversol, isomalt, malted barley, maltodextrin, malts, mannitol, nectars, pentose, raisin syrup, ribose, rice malt, rice syrup, rice syrup solids, sorbitol, sorghum, sucanat, sucanet, xylitol, xylose

Sugar Faux Pas

Don't get fooled by products that are labeled "sugar-free." Sugar is often replaced with sugar alcohols or artificial sweeteners. Remember to always read the ingredients. You can use the sidebar on page 60 as a guide for identifying sneaky sugars.

Sweet Supplements

Occasionally I'll let a little sugar alcohol or stevia use slide for clients, but that's only when the good outweighs the bad. That's the case with some supplements, even ones I recommend like my favorite magnesium supplement, which include small amounts of sugar alcohol or stevia to make them more palatable. This is the only time I say sweetener is OK, because it appears in something you can't overeat and it doesn't have a direct influence on your taste buds or cause cravings.

were 30 percent more likely to have some type of cardiovascular event and 50 percent more likely to die from heart disease than women who drank no diet soda.

I recommend that you stay away from even the more natural sweeteners, like stevia, when it comes to your food choices. We just don't need food to be that sweet. These artificial sweeteners bombard our taste buds with heavy-duty sugary sensations. Over time, we lose the ability to actually taste small amounts of sugar because we've had our sugar senses dulled. Take a break from added sugar and fully nix artificial sweeteners and soda—then see what you notice after three days!

While artificial sweeteners and sodas are nonnegotiable, there are some other items that I would prefer you avoid, but they aren't as much of a deal breaker. These include dried fruit and juice. Both of these options can vary, depending on the brand or the type, from a healthy food to a sugar bomb. Using a few dates to naturally sweeten your smoothie is one thing. Using sugary dried cranberries in your salad is another. When it comes to dried fruit, make sure that there is no additional sugar added (read the ingredients—do I sound like a broken record yet?) and try to use it only in a pinch or when it's in one of the approved bars.

Juice is another hit-or-miss option. I love a good green vegetable juice. It's loaded with vitamins and nutrients, and it's the one food choice in which the lack of protein and fiber is a good thing, because the juice gets absorbed quickly, as does all the nutrition. When I talk about green juices, I'm talking about juice that is primarily made with greens and vegetables and has only a small amount of fruit in it. My ideal juice recipe is all veggies, mainly green ones, plus one low-sugar fruit like an apple. Lemon or lime can be a bonus ingredient too. If you want to drink any other kind of juice, it goes into the intentional indulgence category, and in all honesty, I'd much rather splurge on something more worth it than orange or apple juice. But that's your call. At the end of the day, if you can cut back on your sugar intake by any amount, you're going to be doing great things for your body. I don't like to give a maximum amount of sugar to eat per day because it's not how we eat food. If you follow the sugar rules and stop sweetening things, opt for plain or unsweetened food choices, and read the ingredients, then your sugar intake is already going to be lower than it was. Then, if you want to make room for a sweet intentional indulgence (as we'll discuss in the next section), just go for it. That's the way to have your cake and eat it too.

Q. If I never eat dessert, do I still need to worry about sugar?

A. Sugar isn't reserved for sweet foods. Many clients tell me they don't have a sweet tooth, but then I see that their favorite foods are pizza, bagels, and pasta, all of which are just sugar in a savory form. Don't let the salty taste fool you—white flour is a dessert in savory clothing.

 Rule #5 Summary

Dramatically reduce your sugar intake by simply not adding sugar to your drinks, coffee, yogurt, and/or oatmeal; opting for plain or unsweetened options whenever possible; and reading the ingredients of store-bought items to make sure sneaky sugar isn't hiding there.

Rule #6
Indulge Intentionally

This is my favorite rule for numerous reasons. I love seeing the surprise on my clients' faces when I tell them there is room in their diet for something they had previously considered to be gone from their lives for good. Many people have a misconception of what a diet really is and are used to incredible restrictions with no wiggle room. Are you actually dieting if you get to eat a cookie or a slice of pizza? That's why the whole notion of a diet doesn't make any sense, because you can't avoid everything forever.

It's true, even on the Diet Detox you can't eat everything in front of you. But what makes this diet so effective and user-friendly is that here is a place on your plate for almost every food. Let's use one of my favorite clients as an example here.

Amy had been my client for four months. She had lost over 20 pounds and was following the rules. Each session when Amy came in, I noticed that her food diary was really good, almost too good. She ate a piece of dark chocolate daily, but not a fry or a speck of white flour. While this is great in some ways, in other ways it's a setup for failure.

I told Amy that I wanted her to have a weekly intentional indulgence, but when I checked her food diary after another week, she hadn't done it. I asked her why she wasn't letting herself have the occasional treat, and she replied that she was worried that if she started indulging, she wouldn't be able stop, and that the indulgence would derail all her hard work.

While Amy's fears are justified, this scenario is exactly what an intentional indulgence is supposed to help you avoid. When we eat foods that we've given ourselves permission to eat, we tend to eat them in appropriate amounts (note that I didn't say "in moderation"—that terms just bugs me!). On the contrary, when we eat foods that we've labeled "forbidden" or "not part of the diet plan," that's when we overdo it. Who hasn't eaten something on the "bad" list and then said, "Well, I've already messed up, so I might as well keep going"? Who hasn't said, "I've just blown the day with my eating, so I might as well just keep eating more and start again fresh tomorrow"? And here you are once more in a yo-yo dieting pattern that leads to more weight gain at the end of the day. What I've discovered in my practice is that feeling guilty about your food choices leads you to make additional poor food choices. It's a cyclical pattern. The worse you feel about yourself, the worse your food choices will be, leading you to feel poorly about yourself, then leading you to make another poor food choice, and so on. So basically any restrictive diet is setting you up to fail. That's the beauty of an intentional indulgence, or giving yourself the permission to eat something off-label so to speak—it takes away the guilt. By removing the guilt, we lose the need to overeat and feel poorly about the food choice that was made. An intentional

> *"The Diet Detox has repaired my relationship with food. I now know what it is like to enjoy food and use it to properly fuel my body. I never question my eating anymore because I know what to put on my plate. I just follow the rules and enjoy the nutritious and tasty food options."*
>
> —Melissa S., teacher

indulgence is empowering. An intentional indulgence is a planned food choice that isn't a regular part of your healthy eating plan. I allow it once a week in this program. This isn't the same as a cheat day. Lots of people asked me if they could eat well during the week and then cheat on the weekends. Cheat days are just a short-term diet cycle with a more fun label and, like any on/off diet does, they set you up for failure.

Once I finally got Amy to understand the importance of these indulgences, we got right to work talking about what she's truly craving. This is a really fun part of my job! I asked her what her favorite indulgence was and, after thinking about it for a while, she said the truffle French fries at a local restaurant called Flex Mussels. (For the record, I've had them and they're fantastic!)

Amy and I made a plan. She made a reservation for her next dinner out and was going to order the truffle fries. My rules were that she, not her friend or husband, had to be the one to order them from the waiter; she could share them if she wished; and she could eat as many as she wanted.

The following week when Amy came in, I took a look at her food diary. Ironically enough, the days leading up to her intentional indulgence were extra clean. When I asked her why, she told me that she was so excited for the fries that any other indulgent bites just weren't worth it to her. The fries were written in pink in her diary and she told

"I found the Diet Detox and from page one it clicked. I liked Brooke's frank way of speaking and needed that step-by-step guidance she provided. Knowing there was really no end to this plan was a little nerve-racking at first, but then I realized that for all these years my problem has been starting and stopping diets. This new perspective has led me to shed 40-plus pounds! I don't feel deprived, I know when I can indulge, and I never feel guilty about what I eat. It is amazing what you can accomplish by going on the Diet Detox."

—V.L., professor

me that they were delicious—and that she only ate half of them. In the past, Amy would have eaten the entire serving and then felt guilty about it and would then opt for dessert since the dinner was a diet bust. When I inquired why she didn't finish the serving, she told me that by the time she was halfway through, she wasn't as interested anymore. They tasted amazing in the beginning, and then once they were no longer incredibly delicious, she didn't want another one. She told me they sat next to her while she finished her dinner and she wasn't even tempted to eat more. It's really amazing what simple internal permission can do for your self-control.

When I talk about nutrition for kids, I often tell parents that if you put food on a pedestal, then it stays on a pedestal. What I mean by this is that if you are constantly dangling a cookie in front of your kid as a reward or a super-special treat, the obsession for it is only going to grow stronger. When something special is actually within reach, then it loses some of its specialness. If you're a parent, try to leave a plate of cookies out in front of your kids. On the first day they'll likely eat too many, on the second day they'll eat fewer, and on the third day they will hardly touch them. The same thing happens for us adults. When these French fries were no longer forbidden to Amy, she was able to eat some and move on. It's almost like the more exposure you have to a certain food, the less reactive you are to it.

While I'm not a fan of the Weight Watchers points system, one component that I think is really smart is allowing for almost any food to fit into a diet plan. That said, I've still seen the system abused. For example, some people eat lettuce all day so they can have a binge-worthy meal for dinner. That's just setting yourself up for failure and yo-yoing.

What I truly love about the intentional indulgence concept (aside from that cookie I ate while writing this chapter!) is that it helps you weed out the delicious foods from the not-worth-it foods, all while allowing you to eat something guilt-free. That said, I still have some ground rules for it.

1. An Intentional Indulgence Must Be Planned Ahead

This is the whole point. Make it *intentional*. A planned treat rather than an unplanned one is how you set yourself up for success rather than failure. Think about what food would taste amazing or what you might be missing or craving. Then figure out where the best place to get it will be or when you're going to make it at home. Since having an intentional indulgence every day wouldn't do you any favors on the scale, aim for once a week. Really give some thought to what next week's treat is going to be.

2. You Cannot Feel Any Guilt About Eating It

Guilt leads to weight gain, plain and simple. If you're going to feel guilty about the indulgence, then either you haven't set yourself up properly or you're opting for the wrong choice. Some people need baby steps to work up to a proper indulgence after so many years of restriction and bingeing. A client of mine couldn't be near a bag of potato chips without overeating them, so I had her buy the small snack size to start with once a week. After a month, she was able to have healthy amounts for her intentional indulgence without overdoing it. Start small if you have some anxiety about the indulgence, and then prove to yourself that it will not ruin all your hard work or push you over the edge.

3. Make It Worth It

Don't blow the chance to eat something crave-worthy by taking a few bites of someone else's dessert. If it wasn't good enough for you to order on your own, then it's likely not worth indulging in.

4. Be Smart

While indulging is something I recommend, it's still not a free pass to the nonnegotiables. Don't use your intentional indulgence on chemical-filled candy or soda. This is the chance to eat something *good*. You want a cookie? Bake it yourself or go to a bakery—don't get it from a package. You want ice cream? Eat proper ice cream made with real eggs, milk, and sugar, not mystery-ingredient frozen yogurt. Also, remember to balance it all out. Want pizza? Have it (a slice or two) with a large salad. Want dessert? Eat a great protein- and fiber-filled meal beforehand.

5. Replace Your Starch

Give up one starch for an intentional indulgence. Clearly a slice of whole-grain bread or a banana is better than a cookie or a slice of pizza when it comes to losing weight, but this system of substituting will add balance to what you're eating for the rest of the day.

When you take the first bite of your intentional indulgence, confirm with yourself that it's delicious and worth it, and that you'll feel no guilt. If the answer is yes to all those questions, then enjoy every bite you want to take. If your companions question why you're eating pizza, fries, or cake on a diet—tell them your nutritionist told you to do it.

 Rule #6 Summary

Each week, plan your intentional indulgence ahead of time. Make sure it's worth it and you don't feel any guilt about it. Opt for real food rather than highly processed food, and skip a starch that day to help balance the rest of your meals.

Rule #7
Supplement Smartly

It would be amazing if we all lived and ate well enough to meet the nutritional demands of our bodies. But that's just not the case. Even those who eat the most well-rounded diets are still most likely missing certain nutrients that are either hard to find in food or nearly impossible to eat enough of to meet the recommended amounts.

The challenge with taking supplements is that the store aisles are overwhelming when it comes to picking out which vitamin, mineral, or antioxidant you should purchase. I spend hours of my time reading about new products, spend days walking through convention centers meeting with brand representatives, and regularly use myself as a guinea pig to try out supplements. So I went ahead and did the hard work for you and have listed the supplements that I recommend. I'm especially excited about a lot of the options listed here because I got to work on them behind the scenes and help create the exact products I thought were missing from the marketplace. (These are marked with a *.) All the products in this chapter meet my criteria: they are not insanely expensive, they are easy to find either at stores or online, and they are brands that I support and work with or know well. They also all have solid science behind them and meet the stringent standards that I look for in any supplement, food, or product.

So the important question is, what should you be taking? I break these supplements into two groups: The first group is what I recommend for most people across the board, as long as they don't have any health conditions to contraindicate a particular supplement (be sure to check with your primary caregiver); I call these the "essentials." The second group is for those who want to take a further step into total wellness or perhaps need a little extra help with something like sleep, muscle recovery, relaxation, or even losing weight; that's my "bonus" group.

Essentials

Fiber Supplement

Brand Recommendation: FibeHER by Reserveage*

This isn't your grandmother's Metamucil. As you know by now, there are numerous benefits of fiber. That's why I was excited to help create a fiber supplement that adds not only extra fiber (8 grams per serving) to your day, but also extra protein, so you have Rule #1 in the most convenient method ever. The specific fiber, called Fibersol-2, that we use in this formula has been extensively studied for over 25 years. When taken with a meal, this fiber can help keep your heart healthy and help maintain healthy blood triglyceride levels. As fiber does, this supplement also helps maintain blood sugar levels and control the insulin response that happens after eating. This is always my goal for every meal, so there is even more reason for me to recommend that you take this supplement before breakfast. When your blood sugar levels are stable, losing weight and maintaining your weight loss are much easier.

The proteins that are in FibeHER help keep you full and satisfied. One of the protein sources is Verisol, a high-quality hydrolyzed collagen that is easily digestible and great for your body; it is also non-GMO and nonallergenic. Even more, this specific collagen has been shown in studies to reduce wrinkles and improve skin elasticity—bonus!

Since the switch to the Kick-Starter program can be tough, I highly recommend taking FibeHER every morning before breakfast. It gives you a bit of an edge to help you follow the plan. (For even more of an edge, check out Provance or Fit Kick in the "Bonus Supplements" section on page 80.) Even after you complete the Kick-Starter program, taking a daily fiber supplement that also provides protein will be beneficial for your health in the long run. It will help you maintain your weight loss, stabilize your blood sugar levels, stay regular when using the bathroom, and please your doctor with your cholesterol numbers. What's not to love?

Omega-3 Fatty Acids

Brand Recommendation: Ultimate Omega 2X Mini by Nordic Naturals

Omega-3 fatty acids are recommended by many physicians, and it is one of the foundational supplements that I routinely recommend in my practice. Omega-3 fatty acids are found in fatty fish, like salmon, sardines, oysters, and tuna, which should be part of your diet on the Diet Detox anyway. But even if you're eating fish regularly (two to three times per week), it's hard to know if you're getting enough omega-3 fatty acids to meet your needs. If you don't eat fatty fish regularly or at all, then you should absolutely take this supplement.

There are three main types of omega-3 fatty acids: eicosapentae-noic acid (EPA), docosahexaenoic acid (DHA), and alpha-linolenic acid (ALA). Both EPA and DHA are mainly found in seafood, especially fatty fish and sea vegetables like algae. ALA is the most common form of omega-3 fatty acids that we get through our diet, but it's not easy for the body to convert ALA to EPA or DHA, which is how the body can best use these fatty acids. That's why it's important to supplement with EPA and DHA specifically.

Omega-3 fatty acids have been shown to help with many conditions, including heart disease, skin issues, depression, anxiety, and poor sleep. The science behind omegas and mood disorders like depression and anxi-ety is kind of awesome. In one study, supplementing with EPA had the same benefits as using Prozac, and combining the two had incredible benefits in subjects with depression. Omega-3 intake can also reduce the risk of Alzheimer's disease, dementia, and other age-contributing men-tal decline. Omega's benefits for heart disease are also constantly being researched. Omega-3 fatty acids have been studied for their ability to lower triglyceride levels, lower blood pressure, increase HDL (the good cholesterol), and even reduce the plaque that can harden the arteries— something we'd certainly like to avoid!

We will talk about sleep and its importance to your health and weight in the section on Rule #8 (see page 84). While I will later recommend some supplements to help you with this specifically, omega-3 can also be beneficial for sleep. Low levels of DHA have been linked to low levels of melatonin, a hormone that tells your body it's time to fall asleep. Studies have shown that supplementing with omegas can improve the length and the quality of sleep in adults.

Some omegas are not so fun to take because they leave you with an unpleasant taste in your mouth—you're literally burping fish. No, thank you. The brand I recommend here is on the smaller side compared to most omega supplements. That, along with its lack of gross aftertaste, is one of the reasons I recommend this specific product. If the pill form isn't your thing, there are liquid forms too. Either way, pill or liquid, this supplement is among the essentials.

The New Multivitamin

Brand Recommendation: Nightly One by Twinlab*

As I've said, I find most multivitamins to be antiquated. They're loaded with tons of vitamins and minerals that are super-easy to get from a basic diet, yet deficient in key nutrients that they should be providing. That's why I was so excited to help create this multivitamin; it really focuses on the nutrients that are necessary. What's extra-smart here (I wish I could take the credit for it, but I can't) is that this multivitamin is to be taken before bed. That's because it's designed in two specific ways: some of the nutrients help set you up for a good night's sleep, and many of the other nutrients are best absorbed when your body is at rest. Thus the supplement is especially effective because it optimizes your evening hormone activity. It basically benefits from changes in your body at night. So what's in this nightly multivitamin?

Magnesium

I've been referring to magnesium as the next vitamin D lately because we're finally recognizing how important this mineral is. Not to mention that we're also becoming aware of just how many people are deficient in magnesium. Studies suggest that more than half of the population in the United States isn't meeting its magnesium needs.

Q. Can I just eat my kids' gummy vitamins and call it a day?

A. The short answer: no. I shouldn't even have to write more than this, but I will. First, I am not a fan of gummy vitamins, even the ones formulated for adults. Why? Because you're an adult (though I get the appeal). Second, as I've mentioned, I think most multivitamins are antiquated and are missing many important nutrients that our bodies depend on. So skip your kids' vitamins and take a look at the supplements listed in this chapter, which I recommend to all my clients.

And magnesium deficiency can lead to basically everything you don't want: it can cause muscle cramping, migraines, heart arrhythmias, restless leg syndrome, constipation, and blood sugar issues—should I continue?

Nothing good happens with too little magnesium. Your body needs magnesium to function properly. Over 300 enzymes in the body depend on magnesium to work effectively. These enzymes are in turn needed by your DNA and, for those who can remember high school science, ATP, which basically allows our cells to use energy. Every single cell in your body needs magnesium to function. Magnesium is also crucial for helping your body handle stress. When you're stressed or have a stressful event, your body releases cortisol and adrenaline to react to the stress, creating that fight-or-flight reaction we all know about. But what happens afterwards? That's when magnesium kicks in to bring you back to baseline and help your body basically chill out.

Speaking of chilling out, magnesium is a natural relaxant for your body, which means it's a great mineral to have in the evening to set you up for a good night's sleep. I talk more about ways to set yourself up for a good night's sleep in in the section on Rule #8 (see page 84). As you'll find out, I take sleep really seriously; don't mess with me before bedtime! In my office I use the term "sleep foreplay" to refer to the steps you take to set the mood for a good night's rest. Taking a vitamin with magnesium before bed is one of those steps. Gamma-aminobutyric acid (GABA) neurotransmitters are a calming system we have that tells our brain to shut down for a bit. Without GABA, our minds race back to our to-do lists, strange conversations we had that day, and other unhelpful thoughts. Or if you're like me, random TV theme songs. Magnesium is vital for GABA to do its job so that you can go to sleep and do your job the next day.

Foods rich in magnesium are dark leafy greens, nuts, avocados, dark chocolate (bonus!), and dried fruit. But even with all these options, it's hard to meet our magnesium needs because our bodies lose magnesium every day just by getting up and functioning.

Vitamin D

This vitamin became trendy over the last few years, and for good reason. Many people are deficient, which is a big deal as adequate levels of vitamin D are necessary for our bodies to function properly. Studies have shown that vitamin D is required for both maintaining a healthy heart and preventing a heart attack. There is even interesting evidence that vitamin D prevents the flu and helps the immune system.

That said, vitamin D, which is actually more like a hormone than a vitamin, is hard to find in food. The best sources of vitamin D are cod liver oil, salmon, mackerel, tuna, sardines, and raw milk. Hence we need to supplement. There are two main forms of this vitamin, D3 and D2. D3, the animal form of vitamin D, has a better effect on blood levels of vitamin D than does D2, the plant form. This means that supplementing with vitamin D3 will have a better impact on your blood levels than supplementing with D2. That's why I recommend supplementing daily with vitamin D3.

L-Theanine

L-theanine is an amino acid that's not talked about enough. It's found mainly in teas and promotes both mental and physical relaxation without causing drowsiness. It can also help improve quality of sleep and boost concentration. The effect, often referred to as "alert calmness," comes from its influence on neurotransmitters.

Vitamin B12

Your body goes into repair mode at night, and that's why it's so important to have vitamin B12 before you go to sleep. Vitamin B12 is needed for nightly cell repair and has been shown to influence the release of melatonin to help your body naturally get into that sleepy state.

Zinc

Zinc supports your immune system and the immune functions that are mobilizing during sleep. It's basically the nighttime wingman to your hardworking immune system.

And More

There's a lot more in this multivitamin, but although you take it at night, I don't want to put you to sleep while reading this. There are nutrients like vitamin B6, choline, selenium (which fights inflammation amongst other things), and pyrroloquinoline quinone (PQQ) (which supports brain health and function). Plus a small dose of melatonin (1 milligram), which is safe for daily use and helps your body prepare to get some much-needed R&R.

Probiotic

Brand Recommendation: Beautiflora by Reserveage*

It shouldn't be news by now that probiotics are good for you. In fact, I've been recommending them for years. The main concept is that our center of health is basically located in our gut, right in our intestines. Sexy, right? What was originally thought to be connected only to digestive and belly health has now been linked to heart health, brain heath, immune system function, and even weight issues. The newest research is connecting the type of bacteria that we have in our gut—or our microbiome—to our weight. Some types of gut bacteria are more common in thinner people and others are more common in heavier people—this, of course, is fascinating to me. Bacteroidetes are more common in lean people all over the world. These bacteria love fiber and thrive on a healthy diet. Firmicutes are more populous in heavier people and love to feed on sugar and simple carbohydrates. So how do you get the best type of bacteria in your gut so you can benefit in every way possible?

Happy Gut

Not only is the Diet Detox designed to keep you happy, but it's also designed to keep your gut bacteria happy. Tons of fiber and very little sugar will make your gut a happy home for lean bacteria.

The first step is to set up an environment in your gut where the bacteria can thrive—this is the step that's often skipped. To do this, you need to feed your bacteria with prebiotics. That's what's so smart about Beautiflora. It contains the healthy prebiotic PreticX, which provides a buffet that bacteroidetes (aka skinny bacteria) love to eat, and the probiotic blend LeanSpore; both of these create an optimal environment for a healthy gut.

The next important step to a healthy, skinny gut is to make sure you have the right type of bacteria in your gut to eat the prebiotics. That's where probiotics, or live culture bacteria, come in. There are tons of probiotics, some with billions of colony-forming units (CFUs) and tons of different strains. The problem with these probiotics is that you can never guarantee that they are still active (technically the term should be "alive," but that word just creeps me out here) by the time you take your pill. Even if you take a pill that's still "active," the digestion process is a rough trip, and due to the unpleasant conditions of your gastrointestinal tract, the bacteria might not survive to make it to your intestines, where they need to set up shop.

That's where the spores that are in this product come in. I am predicting that spores are the future of probiotics, and I totally geeked out over the research and science behind their potential. When I realized we were able to combine spores and prebiotics in one single supplement, my mind was blown! Now let's get back to why spores rule. Spores are basically probiotic seeds wrapped in heavy-duty armor, plus they're almost asleep and resting (that is, they're dormant). So not only do they survive packaging and transit until they arrive in your bathroom cabinet, but they have this great protection so that after they're ingested they can survive digestion until they reach the place where they belong. They also have the ability to completely change over the bacteria in your gut to the healthy guys, because once they reach your intestines, they germinate and colonize. They take over but in a good way!

There's a process called "metabolic reconditioning," which is basically a metabolism makeover, and these spores can do it. When they are set up in the right environment (hello, prebiotics), they help create these cool fat-killing compounds called short-chain fatty acids (SCFAs). SCFAs basically control your metabolism, so the more SCFAs, the better. The bacteria in the specific spores in Beautiflora have been shown to increase production of SCFAs by 40 percent. They're basically reconditioning your metabolism to be a lean, mean, fat-burning machine.

Bonus Supplements

Diet Support

Brand Recommendations: Provance by Rebody* or Fit Kick by Twinlab*

Bear with me here; I'm not promoting a diet pill, so let's just get that right out of the way. I promote healthy eating and smart choices. But making those smart choices isn't always easy, and I have found after many years of practice that when people start seeing the number on the scale going in the right direction, they find it much easier to continue to make smart choices. So I like to offer some hand-holding for people who may need that extra boost. Either of these products provide that support.

Provance and Fit Kick are totally safe, natural, stimulant- and caffeine-free supplements containing clinically tested Slimvance, which is made from three ancient herbs, turmeric (*Curcuma longa*), drumstick leaves (*Moringa oleifera*), and curry leaves (*Murraya koenigii*). That's it.

So what do these supplements do? The combination of herbs, two of which are always in my kitchen spice cabinet, helps prevent fat from accumulating, helps the body more efficiently break down fat cells (a process called lipolysis), and directly affects weight.

The studies behind these products show that they can help you see results in as little as two weeks. I like them as an extra support for the Kick-Starter program. Stay on one of them for about a month to help keep you motivated and give you extra support until you feel fully "fluent" in the Diet Detox.

Sleep Helper

Brand Recommendation: Dreamory by Twinlab*

I'll admit that I'm obsessed with sleep. The truth is, a good night's sleep can make the difference between a good day and a bad day. The evening multivitamin that I recommend, Nightly One, will help you get ready for sleep, but for those who still find sleep elusive, I recommend Dreamory. As I mentioned earlier, gamma-aminobutyric acid (GABA) is an amino acid in our body that functions as a calming neurotransmitter in our central nervous system. Healthy people who have insomnia are often found to have reduced levels of GABA. Traditional sleeping pills/aids don't actually contain GABA, but they help GABA work better in the body. However, these sleeping pills have many unpleasant side effects, so I always prefer to offer a natural alternative. Low levels of GABA in the body also cause frequent awakening throughout the night—hence Dreamory. This supplement works by helping the brain shut down for bedtime—it's calming and then some. Many studies have shown that not only does GABA work quickly as a natural relaxant but it also reduces anxiety and can help boost immunity during times of stress.

Extra Magnesium

Brand Recommendation: Natural Calm by Natural Vitality

As I talked about in the section on the multivitamin, Nightly One, I'm a big fan of magnesium and its role in the body. Sometimes we all need a little extra magnesium, and this supplement is the way to go. I like to recommend this powdered supplement for periods of stress or times when your body is overworked. When I see clients working like crazy to meet deadlines, college students pulling all-nighters during finals, or my med school students working 24-hour shifts, I tell them to take this supplement at night. Since this also helps muscles recover from tough physical exertion, I also recommend it to athletes to help their bodies dispose of lactic acid buildup. Studies have also shown that magnesium supplements can help boost performance in athletes and help them cope with the physical stress of their workouts or competitions.

When you use this product, it helps relax your mind so you can sleep well, chills out your muscles to help them recover from your workout or a physical strain, and relaxes your digestive system if you're feeling backed up. I like to take it before bed, drinking it in a cup of tea, and then set the mood for a good night's sleep. Magnesium really is the ultimate chill pill.

Blue Light Protection: Lutein and Zeaxanthin

Brand Recommendation: Ocuguard Blutein Protection by Twinlab

I've been quite clear on the importance of sleep throughout this whole book. The more I learn about blue light and the effect it can have on our sleep, the more I want to learn. We look at blue light all the time now. Between our phones, TVs, computers, and even the lights used in our homes and offices, we're constantly being exposed to blue light. In fact, a widely respected internet analyst, Mary Meeker, estimates that Americans spend an average of 444 minutes a day looking at screens—that's over 7 hours a day. The problem is twofold: blue lights keep us awake and they are damaging to our eyes. I've recently noticed a third dimension of this problem in some of my clients. They get eye fatigue during the day while working but mistake this eye fatigue for hunger; they then have extra snacks either as an excuse to take a break from the computer or as a treat to keep them going through this fatigue.

While I can't get everyone off his or her screen, we can do something about the damage that is being caused by blue light. In the sleep section (see Rule #8 on page 84), I mention that some smartphones have a blue-light-blocking night option, and I'd love it if you kept that on all day.

There are also glasses you can wear to help decrease your exposure on a daily basis. They may not be super-fashionable, but they are effective.

As a dietitian, what concerns me about blue light exposure—in addition to the overeating and sleep issues (as if those weren't enough)—is the drop in phytonutrient levels associated with increased exposure. Phytonutrients protect our retinas from damage and have health-protecting qualities. Our eye health depends on two specific phytonutrients called lutein and zeaxanthin, which are found inside our eyes. We can't make these compounds on our own, so our bodies depend on our diet and supplements to provide them for us. That's why I recommend Ocuguard Blutein Protection for anyone who is concerned about eye health, has a lot of blue screen exposure (as I have while writing this book), or gets really tired around 3:00 PM and reaches for unhealthy snacks (as I'm tempted to do right now).

The phytonutrients in this supplement have been connected to improvements in eye health, brain health, skin health, sleep quality, and the body's reaction to stress. If you're at a screen regularly, travel often (airports have lots of blue light), or just find your eyes getting tired frequently, then this is a supplement designed to help you.

Rule #7 Summary

Supplement daily with the four essentials: **FibeHER, Ultimate Omega 2X Mini, Nightly One**, and **Beautiflora**. If you need bonus supplements, boost your health with **Provance** or **Fit Kick**; **Dreamory**; **Natural Calm**; and/or **Ocuguard Blutein Protection**.

Rule #8
Get Some Sleep

Clients are often surprised when I ask about their habits beyond the foods they eat and their exercise routine. Often my questions regarding sleep habits catch them off guard, as they assume we'll be talking only about food. The reason I want to know about sleep habits is that I find that they generally indicate how well people take care of themselves. Often when I help my clients fix their poor sleeping habits, the rest of their diet plan comes together more quickly. But sleep is also the area where I get the most pushback. I find it kind of hilarious that I can get clients to give up artificial sweeteners or even booze, but they are much more resistant if I ask them to go to bed a little earlier. Many scientific studies show a connection between sleep—or lack of sleep—and weight and health issues. In a study published in the *American Journal of Clinical Nutrition*, researchers found a connection between lack of sleep and an increased risk of obesity. And a meta-analysis (a review of numerous studies) published in the journal *Sleep* showed that shorter sleepers, both adults and children, had a greater risk of obesity than longer sleepers. There's even a link between lack of sleep and risk for type 2 diabetes. In other research published in *Annals of Internal Medicine*, scientists discovered that women who slept 5 hours or less at night were more likely to develop diabetes than women who slept for at least 7 hours at night. Sleep deprivation over a period of time can lower insulin sensitivity, making you more at risk for insulin resistance, which leads to metabolic syndrome. Ready to hit the sack yet? There's more. There is a hormone in our body called leptin that is known as a satiety hormone and helps regulate appetite. Researchers at Stanford University School of Medicine found a connection between sleep deprivation and low leptin levels. This makes sense because many people tend to reach for those extra bites or extra carbs when they are sleep-deprived.

As for the ideal times to go to bed and wake up, I can be flexible. I'm generally a fan of "early to bed, early to rise," but the most important things are that you get enough sleep and that you're consistent. A consistent sleep pattern sets the tone for your body's hormones to ebb and flow in the most productive way. Lack of sleep is stressful on the body, and stress can lead to the buildup of another hormone, cortisol, which can

Case Study: Susan

Susan is a successful psychologist. She was always able to maintain her weight, but over the last two years she's gained about 15 pounds. When she came to me, she said her eating habits hadn't changed much and her exercise routine was still the same. When we compared her past and present life, we noticed that the only difference was that her youngest child had gone to college, so she was now an empty nester. The more we talked, the more I realized that in this situation it was less about the food and more about the lifestyle. In going over her food diary and her typical "day in the life," I saw that the factor that varied the most was her sleep habits. Since she no longer needed to wake up early to get her kids to school, Susan had starting staying up late on occasion and sleeping in when she didn't have an early patient—and had basically lost all consistency in her sleeping routine. She also had a new habit of drinking a glass of wine every night.

Once we got her eating fully set up and mapped out, I wanted to tackle the sleep. I first asked about the glass of wine at night. Now let me say this quickly: I am pro-booze. I have two kids and run my own business, so I totally get the need to have a drink. And I respect people who choose to drink, but from a weight loss perspective, booze not only lets the pounds creep up but also affects your quality of sleep. When I brought this up with Susan, she said that the wine was a treat and that it helped her fall asleep. She really pushed back on changing her bedtime and said that she enjoyed being on her own schedule after spending so much time on her children's. I then pushed back because that is what I do. I stressed to her that if she wanted to lose the stubborn weight, she had to give these changes a shot. We eliminated the weeknight drinking and came up with structured bedtimes and wake times to give her day a little bit of a boost. Within two weeks of cutting back on the booze and following structured sleep suggestions, Susan had dropped 5 pounds. She was now sleeping from 10:00 PM to 6:00 or 7:00 AM most nights and found that a lot of her snacking, which had been happening all day long, was gone.

cause sleeplessness. In periods of stress, we produce more of this hormone, which makes it more difficult to sleep, which leads to more cortisol production. This is a vicious cycle, as cortisol is linked to high levels of blood sugar, low insulin sensitivity, and inflammation. Sleep deprivation even affects the way our brain works. At UC Berkeley a team of researchers used brain-imaging scans to show that lack of sleep causes more activity in a certain area of the brain, which is connected with the motivation to eat. So when you are sleep-deprived, it is no longer about willpower—it is literally about brainpower.

In the "Clock Your Meals" section, I mentioned that I wanted to bring back the early-bird special. There are many reasons behind this (aside from my desire to get people to eat with me more frequently). An early dinner gives your body more time to rest prior to falling asleep. This allows your body to digest your dinner while you're still awake instead of while you sleep. If you eat right before bed, you'll have a blood sugar spike and that sugar gets stored as fat, plus it interferes with your sleep quality. That's no good. Eating an early dinner, ideally at least 2 to 4 hours before you hit the hay, allows your body enough time to digest and allows your blood sugar levels to stabilize to help you have a great night's rest. Adding your healthy starch option at your early dinner is also smart for sleeping. According to a report in the *American Journal of Clinical Nutrition*, eating a healthy starch option for an early dinner (4 hours before bed) allows people to fall asleep faster. Who needs that glass of wine anymore?

Setting yourself up for a good night's sleep sets you up for better hormonal balance, healthier brain function, and better food choices. Poor sleep leads to poor food choices, which lead to weight gain, which itself leads to poor sleep. So what can we do to set ourselves up for sleep success? I call this "sleep foreplay," or the steps you need to take to get your body in the mood for a good night of sleep.

1. Lose the booze. You might think that a glass of wine helps you fall asleep more quickly, but you'll miss out on deep and restorative sleep.
2. Eat earlier. Try to eat at least 2 to 4 hours prior to going to bed, if not more.
3. Stick with a consistent bedtime and wake time. This isn't to say you cannot sleep in on the weekends, but consistency is key when it comes to healthy sleep habits.
4. Unplug. Constant blue light exposure from all our electronic devices is affecting our body's biological clock. Try to avoid a screen for at least an hour before bed. At the very least, put down your phones, computers, and iPads as they tend to have the most blue light. Consider

adding the supplement Ocuguard Blutein Protection by Twinlab to help prevent blue light damage and sleep-related issues.

If your smartphone has an option to switch to "night shift," do this whenever possible, especially after 7:00 PM. This cuts down on the amount of blue light produced by your phone. Smartphone, indeed.

5. Supplement smartly with vitamins and minerals that help set up your body for a successful sleep. I recommend Nightly One by Twinlab to set you up for sleep success every night and Dreamory by Twinlab to help you if you're having sleeping issues such as not being able to fall or stay asleep. Read more about these in "Rule #7: Supplement Smartly" on page 73.

 Rule #8 Summary

Aim for a minimum of 7 hours of sleep per night. Set yourself up for a good night of sleep by skipping the booze, eating dinner 2 to 4 hours before bedtime, being consistent with your sleep schedule, avoiding too much blue light exposure, and supplementing smartly.

Rule #9
Drink Water

This is something you know, right? You need to drink water, a solid amount of it, every single day. That's not anything new. But somehow, almost everyone who walks into my office isn't drinking nearly enough on a consistent basis. In fact, *Medical Daily* reported that up to 75 percent of Americans aren't drinking enough, so you're not alone in this.

Bathroom Breaks

As much as I want you drinking water, I don't want it affecting your sleep. Start to "dry out" about 2 to 3 hours before bedtime.

Let's just put this out there clearly: water is the best and most important beverage you should be drinking each day. Plain and simple. I always get hustled by my clients, who try to get me to allow their coffee, tea, or green juices to count toward their water goals. One client even asked if she could drink less water because she ate a lot of fruit. My answer: nope. The truth is that water-rich fruits and vegetables do contribute water to your diet, but I like to use those, plus other caffeine-free beverages, as a bonus. Your ultimate goal should be to get your hydration needs from plain old water.

Why am I such a stickler for water intake? Numerous studies show that water is an effective weight loss tool, especially when consumed before a meal. But beyond the science, I have seen firsthand in my practice the difference in clients when they drink enough water. When my clients start working on consuming more water, I first hear some complaints—the first one is that they have to go to the bathroom all the time and the second one is that it's boring to drink. Neither complaint elicits any sympathy from me. Your bladder will adjust to your water consumption, and boring isn't always a bad thing.

After clients have been on top of drinking enough water for a week or two, they start to experience the positive effects. Some tell me that they're getting compliments on their skin. Others report that their digestive woes went away after a few days of drinking enough water. Still others tell me that they have more energy. All from drinking some boring water.

When water starts to replace other beverages, even better things happen. A study published in the *American Journal of Clinical Nutrition* showed that when water replaced a diet drink (which is a nonnegotiable anyway) after the main meal, there was greater weight reduction during a weight loss program. And it showed that this habit may even improve insulin resistance. This isn't the only study that connected water intake to blood sugar levels. A study published in *Diabetes Care*, the journal for the American Diabetes Association, showed that adults who drank only around half a liter of water per day were more likely to have high blood sugar.

Increased water intake has also been shown to be helpful for weight loss and weight maintenance. The journal *Obesity* published a study in 2015 that investigated whether preloading, or drinking water before a meal, could lead to weight loss for obese patients. The results showed preliminary evidence that this practice works. Another study published in the same journal a few years earlier also suggested that drinking water may promote weight loss in overweight women. This theory is not new, nor is the notion that drinking water is good for you. But time and time again, I see with the thousands of clients in my practice that water intake works for weight loss. Whether it's because drinking water fills you up before a meal, prevents you from mistaking thirst for hunger (that's a big one), or simply reminds you to be healthy, it works. Often when we have small reminders throughout the day that we're trying to be healthy or treat our body right, we tend to continue to make positive choices. The simple act of consciously taking a few extra sips of water forms a healthy connection to how we're treating our body. When we're treating our body well, we then also tend to eat better. It's a healthy positive cycle that literally starts with a glass of water.

So how much water should you be drinking? For clients who are not great water drinkers to begin with, my goal for them is 1.5 liters each day. Then we ultimately increase to 2 liters a day. This isn't a natural change for some people and they often need a little more support. You can

Q. How much water should I drink?

A. Your water goal should be around 2 liters or 64 ounces per day.

put reminders in your calendar to alert you that you need to drink some water every hour. Some of my clients love the apps that are available like WaterMinder. Others buy a new water bottle like a S'well or CamelBak and that's motivating enough—the important thing is to do whatever works for you!

 Rule #9 Summary

Aim for about 2 liters or 64 ounces of water per day. Also, be sure to drink consistently throughout the day rather than all at once.

Rule #10
Exercise

Some of my clients hate asking about this rule when we're in session. The truth is that if you want to reach a healthy weight and maintain that weight, then you are going to need to exercise. Nothing bums me out more than seeing the same people year after year at the gym working out on the elliptical trainer for up to an hour and yet looking no different. A close second is seeing people working out hard and then eating or drinking some nonsense food, like a smoothie made with frozen yogurt, right after they leave the gym. But I digress.

It's my rule that all my clients need to move, somehow. Ideally they are exercising regularly—doing the kind of workout that really makes them sweat, not just coasting on the elliptical (more about this in a bit). And my general rule of thumb is that no more than two days off are allowed. So if you work out on Monday, then skip Tuesday and Wednesday, you must work out again on Thursday. On nonexercise days I still require my clients to move—they need to go for a walk, use the stairs instead of the elevator, stretch, or do whatever they need to do to simply move their body. This helps them remember that they have a body attached to their head—something we could all use a reminder of—and stay mindful of that mind-body connection. Small moments of this awareness are beneficial because when we're more in tune with our body, we tend to feed it better.

Now, on to what I define as exercise. I like a workout that gives you the most bang for your buck—I want you to do something high-intensity and efficient, rather than moderately puttering away for an hour on an elliptical machine or treadmill. I don't mean to denigrate the benefits of going for a walk or doing other low-intensity movements—all of which are important and great for you. But the way I feel about those

Q. I don't really like moving my body, so what exercise can I get the most out of in the least amount of time?

A. You do not need to spend hours in the gym to get results. But I want you to remember that although diet takes the weight off, exercise helps keep it off and also helps shape your body. Just get moving as often as possible, and if you can throw in some interval training with some weights two to three times a week, that is enough to start.

Q. I am obsessed with my spin class—do I need to do anything else?

A. The best kind of exercise is the kind you keep doing. Second best to that is HIIT (high-intensity interval training). So it is great that you love your spin class, but do not forget to give your butt a break and do some weight-bearing exercises too. It will help you speed up your metabolism, control your blood sugar levels, and maintain a healthy weight.

real gym days is like the way I feel about intentional indulgences: if you're going to do it, do it right.

So what's doing it right? It's the kind of workout that challenges your heart, builds lean muscle mass, helps with weight control, and can even help moderate your blood sugar levels. The best of the best for this is called high-intensity interval training (HIIT). I first started researching the effects of HIIT when I was writing *The Sugar Detox*. It was pretty cool to find the specific type of exercise that was most effective in helping control blood sugar levels, not to mention burning fat and building muscle. While the name is intimidating, it's not as scary as it sounds. It's a workout that alternates short periods of intense exercise with short recovery periods. Think of running on a treadmill, but instead of going at your set pace of 6 miles per hour you sprint at 8 miles per hour for 30 seconds every few minutes. These bursts of energy expenditure are more effective for kicking your body into gear. Plus, you don't need to do it for as long to reap the benefits. Just 10 minutes of HIIT a day can do the trick, if you're crunched for time.

I'm not a certified personal trainer, but for some of my clients who are working out without one, I'll often give them an exercise Rx as one of their goals. Together we figure out some interesting ways for them to safely push themselves further while exercising. One of these goals has always been to add intervals to their cardio workout. Originally I just wanted to get them to work harder and to get out of their comfort zone. So when I read the research about HIIT, I knew I was onto something. Any interval training is good for you: it pushes you a bit harder than you'd normally push yourself, so you get better results, and it keeps things more interesting, so you're less likely to get bored while working out. Not only is HIIT effective during the workout, but because of the afterburn effect, it keeps your body working even when you're done with the gym. HIIT can cause an increase in your resting metabolic rate, so you actually can be burning more calories while you're doing nothing. Pretty cool.

HIIT doesn't have to be ultra-high-intensity to be effective either. Interval training is effective at any level, which is why I even recommend it to my clients who are new to working out or perhaps not in the best of shape. Simply walking at a more brisk pace for a minute every few minutes will make your workout do more for you. Any time you can kick up what you're doing a notch, your workout will be that much more worth it and better for your body.

When it comes to trying new methods of exercise, living in New York City really has its perks because there are so many new gyms popping up. A couple of years ago while I was writing *The Sugar Detox*, I came across a boutique gym called the Fhitting Room, which specialized in high-intensity interval training. Of course, I had to test it out. The gym's style of workout had me instantly hooked, from the great instructors to the music. It was a huge challenge, but I saw results. So I asked the Fhitting Room team to create some workouts that I could put in this book, giving everyone access to a great HIIT workout.

There is a nice variety of workouts in these 10 (10!) options for you to choose from. Some require equipment, some do not, some are more difficult than others, and some are shorter than others. Take a look and see what you can do. Aim to incorporate these specific workouts into your gym time at least two days a week, even if it's just sneaking in a quick one. Then use your remaining days of the week to do other forms of cardio or strength training. Just be sure to follow the rule I mentioned earlier: take no more than two days off between workouts and get moving every single day. Also, you can check out my website, b-nutritious.com, or my Facebook page, www.facebook.com/bnutritious/, for even more suggestions about how to just get moving.

 Rule #10 Summary

Move daily and don't skip more than two days between workouts.

10 Workouts by the Fhitting Room

Note: All the recommended weights are a suggestion. Depending on your fitness level and experience with these movements, you may need to adjust your weight. It's important that you choose weights that feel right for you body. Start on the lighter side and work your way up to the recommended weights.

1. 10-Minute Dumbbell Workout

This 10-minute workout will jack your heart rate up in Part 1, making it a great cardio start to your workout while preparing your core, aka your abs and back, for some hard work in Part 2.

Part 1

The first part of this workout is in Tabata format, in which quick periods of activity (20 seconds) are followed by a short period of rest (10 seconds) for a total of 4 minutes. It may not seem challenging at first, but you'll be huffing and puffing pretty quickly.

The Movements

Dumbbell Jacks: Do regular jumping jacks with weights in each hand. Be sure to keep your core strong, especially when raising your arms with the weights over your head.

Dumbbell Sit-Ups: Lie on your back with your arms over your head and hold one dumbbell horizontally between your palms. Start with the dumbbell over your head, then reach for the sky as you sit up.

The Workout

Tabata Workout: Do 4 rounds of these two movements for a total of 4 minutes.

Recommended dumbbell weight: 5 to 10 pounds

   20 seconds Dumbbell Jacks

   10 seconds rest

20 seconds Dumbbell Sit-Ups (1 dumbbell)

10 seconds rest

Recover for 2 minutes before starting part 2.

Part 2

Do the three movements and time yourself for each round. See if you can keep up the same pace each round or even outdo yourself.

The Movements

Dumbbell Alternating Snatches: Stand with your feet slightly wider than shoulder width apart, and place the dumbbell horizontally between the arches of your feet. Bend your knees into a squat position with a flat back, place one hand around the handle of the dumbbell with the palm facing toward you, and explosively lift the dumbbell overhead, trying to keep it as close to your body as possible. Alternate sides with each repetition.

Dumbbell Front Squats: Standing with feet hip width apart, hold a dumbbell in each hand with your elbows bent and the dumbbells by your shoulders. Keep your elbows pointing forward as you squat down. As you start your descent, stick your butt back as if you were sitting down on a chair and push your knees out, while trying to keep your chest up. To complete the movement, squeeze your glutes as you return to the upright position.

Dumbbell Suitcase Walking Lunges: Stand tall holding the dumb-bells in each hand, as if you were holding two suitcases. Begin to do forward walking lunges while maintaining a tall posture. To keep your balance, keep your feet hip width apart. Aim to lightly touch your knee to the ground when you lunge down.

The Workout

Complete the following movements 4 times. Try to move quickly when transitioning between exercises.

Recommended dumbbell weight: 15 to 25 pounds

10 Dumbbell Alternating Snatches

10 Dumbbell Front Squats

10 Dumbbell Suitcase Walking Lunges

2. 15-Minute Dumbbell Workout

This three-part workout is made up of 5-minute AMRAPs (as many rounds as possible). The goal is to see how many rounds of the three exercises you can do in the time allotted. Challenge yourself to beat your previous numbers and see if you can keep the dumbbells in your hands without putting them down between each movement. You'll be feeling this total-body workout in your glutes, quadriceps, and shoulders tomorrow.

Part 1

The Movements

Dumbbell Thrusters: Start with the dumbbells at your shoulders, with your elbows bent and pressed tightly against your body. Squat down as though you're sitting in a chair, and as you come to standing, press the dumbbells up to the ceiling, fully extending your arms overhead. Your legs should really provide the momentum to drive your arms up. This exercise should be done as one continuous fluid movement: you should press up your arms and stand simultaneously.

Dumbbell Alternating Reverse Lunge to Curls: Start with the dumbbells in a suitcase hold, holding one dumbbell in each hand as if you were holding two suitcases. Step backwards with one leg into a reverse lunge. At the bottom of the movement, both knees should be forming a 90-degree angle. The back knee should just touch the floor while the chest stays upright and the shoulders are rolled back. Return to standing and curl the dumbbells to the shoulders.

Dumbbell Squat Thrusts: Stand up straight with arms at your sides and a dumbbell in each hand. Bend at the waist with a slight bend at the knees until the dumbbells reach the floor. Keeping your hands on the dumbbells, shoot your legs out behind you into a plank position, and then jump back. Return to standing with the dumbbells at your sides. The goal is to hold onto the dumbbells throughout the whole movement.

The Workout

5-Minute AMRAP (as many rounds as possible): Complete the following sequence as many times as possible within the 5-minute cap. Try not to stop for rest during the entire 5 minutes. The goal is to complete 4 or more rounds.

Recommended dumbbell weight: 10 to 15 pounds

> 10 Dumbbell Thrusters
>
> 10 Dumbbell Alternating Reverse Lunge to Curls
>
> 10 Dumbbell Squat Thrusts

Part 2

The Movements

Dumbbell Jacks: Do regular jumping jacks with weights in each hand. Be sure to keep your core strong, especially when raising your arms with the weights over your head.

Dumbbell Froggers: Move into a plank position, holding onto your dumbbells, which are on the floor. Jump your feet in to meet your hands, and then jump back out into a plank. Try to keep your butt down throughout the movement. Do this exercise in a continuous, fast motion. If this hurts your palms, eliminate the dumbbells and place your hands on the floor.

Renegade Rows: Start in the push-up position with a wider leg stance to help stabilize your body. Place one dumbbell under each hand. Perform a push-up and bring one dumbbell, then the other, up to your chest, like a row. This is one rep.

The Workout

5-Minute AMRAP (as many rounds as possible): Complete the following sequence as many times as possible within the 5-minute cap. Try not to stop for rest during the entire 5 minutes. The goal is to complete 4 or more rounds.

Recommended dumbbell weight: 10 to 12½ pounds

> 20 Dumbbell Jacks
>
> 8 Dumbbell Froggers with hands on dumbbell
>
> 6 Renegade Rows

Part 3

5-Minute Chipper: A chipper is a set of 5 to 10 movements in which the reps become shorter as you go through the movements. Start with the first exercise and move on to the next one with little or no rest in between. The goal is to complete all movements as quickly as possible and within the 5-minute time cap.

The Movements

Dumbbell Alternating Snatches: Stand with your feet slightly wider than shoulder width apart, and place the dumbbell horizontally between the arches of your feet. Bend your knees into a squat position with a flat back, place one hand around the handle of the dumbbell with the palm facing toward you, and explosively lift the dumbbell overhead, trying to keep it as close to your body as possible. Alternate sides with each repetition.

Dumbbell Russian Twists: Sit on the floor with your knees bent and your feet floating a few inches above the ground (to modify this exercise, keep your feet on the ground for balance). Lean back so your torso is at a 45-degree angle to the floor and your torso and upper legs are in a V shape. Holding one dumbbell in your hands, rotate your torso to one side and then the other side. Keep your back straight, and not rounded, as you rotate.

Man Makers: Start by standing with a dumbbell in each hand at your sides. Bend down, placing the dumbbells in front of you, and jump your feet out to a push-up position with a wider leg stance to help stabilize your body. Perform a push-up, row one dumbbell (bringing it up to your chest and back down), and do the same with the other hand. Jump your feet to the outside of your hands and stand up with the dumbbells by your side. Curl and press the dumbbells overhead to complete one rep.

Push Presses: Holding the dumbbells in the rack position (arms are bent, wrists are straight, elbows are tucked into the rib cage, and dumbbells are at shoulder level), press one dumbbell up directly above your head and completely straighten your arm. Reverse the motion by tucking your elbow back into your rib cage, and then press the other arm vertically up so it's fully straight. In this workout, first do 5 reps with your right arm, and then do 5 reps with your left arm.

The Workout

5-Minute Chipper: Try to complete all the following movements within the allotted 5-minute time.

Recommended dumbbell weight: 15 to 20 pounds

> 30 Dumbbell Alternating Snatches
>
> 20 Dumbbell Russian Twists
>
> 10 Man Makers
>
> 5 Push Presses (right)
>
> 5 Push Presses (left)

3. 10-Minute Kettlebell Workout

A kettlebell is a great conditioning tool that provides a whole-body workout. Using a kettlebell is an effective and efficient way to get both a cardio workout and a strength workout at the same time.

Part 1

The Movements

Jumping Jacks: Do simple jumping jacks, making sure to reach your hands all the way out and above your head.

Air Squats: Stand with your feet hip width apart. Sit back as though you were sitting down in a chair, keeping your chest up. To complete the movement, stand back up and squeeze your glutes as you return to the upright position.

Inchworm to Push-Ups: Stand with your feet hip width apart and bend at the waist, keeping your legs as straight as possible. Reach for your toes and then walk your hands out to a push-up position. This will give your hamstrings a stretch. Once you are all the way out to the plank, perform one push-up (to modify the exercise, drop to your knees) and then walk your hands back toward your feet and stand up to complete one rep.

The Workout

2-Minute Warm-Up: Do each of the following movements for 20 seconds. Complete 2 rounds.

Jumping Jacks

Air Squats

Inchworm to Push-Ups

Part 2

The Movements

Kettlebell Goblet Squats: Stand with your feet a bit wider than hip width, and hold the kettlebell by the handle in front of your chest with your elbows tucked in. Sit back as though sitting down on a chair, keeping your chest up. Be sure to squat below parallel, meaning your hips should fall below your knees. Inhale as you descend and exhale as you come up.

Kettlebell Push Presses: Holding lighter kettlebells, one in each hand, in the rack position (arms are bent, wrists are straight, elbows are tucked into the rib cage, and kettlebells are resting on the bicep and forearm), dip down about 2 inches into a half squat, and then stand up aggressively as you press the kettlebells overhead and straighten your arms. Reverse the motion by tucking your elbows back into your rib cage. Use the momentum of the squat to help you lift the weights up, and challenge yourself to a heavier weight.

Kettlebell Bent-Over Rows: Bend at the waist, keeping a flat back, and then step forward with your left foot and place your left forearm across your left quad. Your upper body should be in a straight line. While keeping your back flat, hold the kettlebell in your right hand, and pull the kettlebell toward your rib cage using your back muscles. Complete all reps on one side, and then reverse the leg and arm positions and complete all reps on the other side.

The Workout

5-Minute Strength Section: Do each of the following movements for 45 seconds, and rest for 15 seconds between exercises. Complete 2 rounds.

Recommended kettlebell weight: 10 to 16 kilograms

Kettlebell Goblet Squats

Kettlebell Push Presses

Kettlebell Bent-Over Rows (left)

Kettlebell Bent-Over Rows (right)

Part 3

A FHIX is a functional high-intensity mix workout. It's a great way to push yourself for the last few minutes of your workout.

The Movements

Kettlebell Swings: Stand with your feet hip width apart, your toes pointed slightly outward, and both hands on one kettlebell. Thrust the bell forward from the hips and swing it to chest level. As the kettlebell comes back down, allow your knees to bend slightly. Now send your butt back and let the momentum take the kettlebell down between your legs/inner thighs, then back to the starting position. That's one rep.

Kettlebell Lunge Pass-Throughs (double count): Stand with the kettlebell in your right hand hanging at your side. Step your left foot into a lunge, dropping the right knee to the floor. Pass the kettlebell under your left leg and into your left hand. Push off your left foot to come back to a standing position. Repeat on the opposite leg. That's one rep.

Kettlebell Plank Reach-Outs (double count): Start in a low plank position on your elbows with your feet wider apart than your shoulders. Make sure your elbows are directly under your shoulders. Alternating hands, reach out in front of you to touch the kettlebell without swaying your hips side to side. Once you have reached out with both your right and your left arms, you have done one rep.

The Workout

3-Minute FHIX (functional high-intensity mix): This workout is an ascending ladder. Start with 2 reps of each movement, and then progress to 4 of each movement, then 6 of each movement. Continue up the ladder for 3 minutes.

Recommended kettlebell weight: 10 to 16 kilograms

Kettlebell Swings

Kettlebell Lunge Pass-Throughs (double count)

Kettlebell Plank Reach-Outs (double count)

4. 15-Minute Kettlebell Workout

Your body has to work a bit harder with kettlebells than with dumbbells because it needs to stabilize more, making this workout more effective than workouts with dumbbells. Your shoulders, aka deltoids, will be feeling this workout for sure!

Part 1

10-Minute Kettlebell Sequence: Do 2 reps of each movement on one side of your body, and then do 2 reps of each movement on the other side. The goal is to complete 5 rounds on both sides within the 10-minute time cap.

The Movements

Kettlebell Dead Cleans: Bend at the waist with one hand grabbing the kettlebell on the floor; the handle should be parallel to you. Keep your back straight, your chest up, and your knees slightly bent. While keeping your chest up, drive to a standing position using the hips and knee extension while rotating the kettlebell around to the rack position (standing straight up, with your arm bent at the elbow and the kettlebell base on the outside of the forearm). Always keep your elbows tucked into your rib cage.

Kettlebell Alternating Reverse Lunges: Start with the kettlebells in a suitcase hold, holding one in each hand as if you were holding two suitcases. Step backwards with one leg into a reverse lunge. At the bottom of the movement, both knees should be forming a 90-degree angle. The back knee should just touch the floor while the chest stays upright and the shoulders are rolled back. Return to standing while engaging your core.

Kettlebell Goblet Squats: Stand with your feet a bit wider than hip width, and hold the kettlebell by the handle in front of your chest with your elbows tucked in. Sit back as though sitting down on a chair, keeping your chest up. Be sure to squat below parallel, meaning your hips should fall below your knees. Inhale as you descend and exhale as you come up.

Kettlebell Strict Presses: Start with the kettlebells in the rack position (standing straight up, with your arm bent at the elbow and the kettlebell base on the outside of the forearm) and press them overhead so that your biceps are alongside your ears and your arms are fully extended. The weight should be challenging, but not so much that you need to use your legs to push the kettlebells overhead. Return to the rack position and repeat.

The Workout

Do 2 reps of each movement on one side of your body, and then do 2 reps of each movement on the other side. The goal is to complete 5 rounds on both sides within the 10-minute time cap.

Recommended kettlebell weight: 8 to 12 kilograms

> Dead Cleans
>
> Alternating Reverse Lunges
>
> Goblet Squats
>
> Strict Presses

Part 2

5-Minute AMRAP (as many rounds as possible): Complete the following sequence as many times as possible within the 5-minute time cap. The goal is to complete 4 to 5 rounds.

The Movements

Kettlebell Goblet Squats: Stand with your feet a bit wider than hip width, and hold the kettlebell by the handle in front of your chest with your elbows tucked in. Sit back as though sitting down on a chair, keeping your chest up. Be sure to squat below parallel, meaning your hips should fall below your knees. Inhale as you descend and exhale as you come up.

Kettlebell Goblet Thrusters: Hold the kettlebell by the handle with both hands in front of your chest and your elbows tucked in. Squat down with your butt back, and then as you come back to standing, press the kettlebell up to the ceiling, fully extending your arms overhead. Your legs should really provide the momentum to drive your arms up; you should press up your arms and stand simultaneously.

Plank Jacks: Start in a low plank position on your elbows, with your elbows under your shoulders, and your feet together. Jump your feet wide and back together. This counts as one rep.

The Workout

5-Minute AMRAP (as many rounds as possible): The goal is to complete 4 to 5 rounds.

Recommended kettlebell weight: 8 to 12 kilograms

5 Goblet Squats

5 Goblet Thrusters

5 Plank Jacks (no kettlebell)

5. 20-Minute Kettlebell Workout

This is a posterior chain workout, which means that it uses all the muscles along the back of your body. In these 20 minutes your calves, hamstrings, glutes, and back will all get a solid workout.

Part 1

The Movements

Air Squats: Stand with your feet hip width apart. Sit back as though you were sitting down on a chair, keeping your chest up. To complete the movement, stand back up and squeeze your glutes as you return to the upright position.

Good Mornings: Stand with your feet hip width apart and your hands behind your head, elbows out. While maintaining a flat back, hinge at the waist and bend over to stretch your hamstrings. Return to standing by squeezing your glutes. It's OK to have a gentle bend in your knees if needed.

Push-Ups: Start in a high plank position with your hands directly under your shoulders. Lower your chest toward the floor, with your back flat and your abs tight, and with your elbows moving back toward your ribs, not out. Then push back up to the starting position to complete one rep. (To modify the exercise, you can do the push-ups with your knees on the floor.)

Mountain Climbers: Start in a high plank position with your hands directly under your shoulders. Alternate driving your right and left knees toward your chest. Keep your hips low and level and your stomach muscles engaged.

2-Minute Body-Weight Warm-Up

Do each movement for 30 seconds and complete 2 rounds.

    Air Squats

    Good Mornings

    Push-Ups

    Mountain Climbers

Part 2

The Movements

Kettlebell Sumo Deadlifts: Start in a wide squat stance with your toes pointed out slightly and the kettlebell on the floor directly in front of you. Squat down with a flat back to pick up the kettlebell and stand up quickly using your glutes. Squat to lower the kettlebell back down. It's great to opt for a heavier kettlebell in this exercise.

Kettlebell Alternating Reverse Lunge to Presses: Start with the kettlebells in the rack position (arms are bent, wrists are straight, elbows are tucked into the rib cage, and dumbbells are at shoulder level) and step backwards into a reverse lunge. At the bottom of the movement, both knees should be forming a 90-degree angle and your back knee should just touch the floor while your chest stays upright. Return to standing as you press the kettlebells overhead.

Kettlebell Swings: Stand with your feet hip width apart, your toes pointed slightly outward, and both hands on one kettlebell. Thrust the bell forward from the hips and swing it to chest level. As the kettlebell comes back down, allow your knees to bend slightly. Now send your butt back and let the momentum take the kettlebell down between your legs/inner thighs, then back to the starting position. That's one rep.

The Workout

Kettlebell "FHITervals": Set up three stations of kettlebells in one straight line. Do each movement for 30 seconds and take 10 seconds to rest; then transition to the next movement. Once you complete all 3 movements, you have completed one round. Do 7 rounds in total.

Recommended kettlebell weight: 6 to 12 kilograms

Station 1: Kettlebell Sumo Deadlifts

Station 2: Alternating Reverse Lunge to Presses

Station 3: Kettlebell Swings

6. 10-Minute Body-Weight Workout

Here is a basic total-body workout that can be done anywhere. There are no excuses that you don't have the equipment, or even the time. I've done this one in a hotel room in pajamas, so truly there are no excuses at all!

The Movements

Reverse Lunges: Start by standing tall with your feet shoulder width apart. Step back into a reverse lunge. At the bottom of the movement, both knees should be forming a 90-degree angle and your back knee should just touch the floor while your chest stays upright. Return to standing and do the movement with the other leg.

Air Squats: Stand with your feet hip width apart. Sit back as though you were sitting down on a chair, keeping your chest up. To complete the movement, stand back up and squeeze your glutes as you return to the upright position.

Froggers: Place your hands on the floor in front of you and jump your feet back into plank position. Jump your feet back to your hands, with your feet landing to the outside of each hand. Try to keep your butt down throughout the movement. Do this exercise in a continuous, fast motion.

Push-Ups: Start in a high plank position with your hands directly under your shoulders. Lower your chest toward the floor, with your back flat and abs tight, and with your elbows moving back toward your ribs, not out. Then push back up to the starting position to complete one rep. (To modify the exercise, you can do the push-ups with your knees on the floor.)

The Workout

Do each movement for 30 seconds. After completing 1 round, take 30 seconds to rest. Complete 4 rounds.

Reverse Lunges

Air Squats

Froggers

Push-Ups

7. 16-Minute Body-Weight Workout

This workout is the next level up from the preceding workout. There are more compound movements, which help make the most of the 16 minutes.

Part 1

The Movements

Air Squats: Stand with your feet hip width apart. Sit back as though you were sitting down on a chair, keeping your chest up. To complete the movement, stand back up and squeeze your glutes as you return to the upright position.

Inchworms: Stand with your feet hip width apart and bend at the waist, keeping your legs as straight as possible. Reach for your toes and then walk your hands out to a push-up position. This will give your hamstrings a stretch. Walk your hands back toward your feet and stand up to complete one rep.

Lateral Lunges: With your feet wide, lunge sideways, pushing your butt back as if you were doing a squat while keeping the other leg straight. Push yourself back into a neutral standing position.

Plank Holds: Start in a push-up position, with your hands directly under your shoulders, your arms straight, your feet close together, and your toes connected with the floor. Engage your stomach muscles to help support you during this hold.

The Workout

Do each movement for 30 seconds and take 10 seconds to transition to the next movement. Complete 2 rounds.

Air Squats

Inchworms

Lateral Lunges (right on the first round, left on the second round)

Plank holds

Recover for 20 seconds before starting the second round.

Part 2

The Movements

Jump Squats: Start in a squat position, with your butt back, your chest up, and your knees behind your toes. From the bottom of the squat, jump up and land back in a squat position. Be sure to land softly to protect your knees. (To modify the exercise, opt for air squats instead; see Part 1.)

Inchworm to Mountain Climbers: Stand with your feet hip width apart and bend at the waist, keeping your legs as straight as possible. Reach for your toes and then walk your hands out to a push-up position. This will give your hamstrings a stretch. Now bring each knee alternately into your chest at a quick pace, while keeping your hips still. Walk your hands back toward your feet and stand up to complete one rep.

Lateral Lunge to Hops (or Balances): With your feet wide, lunge sideways, pushing your butt back as if you were doing a squat while keeping the other leg straight. Push yourself back into a neutral standing position, and then hop at the top of the movement (or modify the exercise by just balancing momentarily on one leg).

Plank-Ups: Start in a low plank position on your elbows, and then move your hands to the positions where your elbows were so you're now up in a high-plank position. Reverse the movement to return to your elbows. This counts as one rep. While doing this, squeeze your glutes, core, and legs to stabilize your hips.

The Workout

Do each movement for 30 seconds and take 10 seconds to transition to the next movement. Complete 2 rounds.

Jump Squats

Inchworm to 4 Mountain Climbers (single count)

Lateral Lunge to Hops (or Balances) (right on the first round, left on the second round)

Plank-Ups

Recover for 20 seconds before starting the second round.

Part 3

The Movements

Broad Jump with 180-Degree Jump Squat Turns: Start with your feet shoulder width apart in a partial squat, and swing your arms back then forward to create momentum to help you jump forward as far as you can. Land in a partial squat and do a jump squat. While you're in the air, turn your entire body around to face the opposite direction.

Inchworm to Mountain Climbers: Stand with your feet hip width apart and bend at the waist, keeping your legs as straight as possible. Reach for your toes and then walk your hands out to a push-up position. This will give your hamstrings a stretch. Now bring each knee alternately into your chest at a quick pace, while keeping your hips still. Walk your hands back toward your feet and stand up to complete one rep.

Lateral Lunge to Reverse Lunge to Front Kicks: With your feet wide, lunge sideways, pushing your butt back as if you were doing a squat while keeping the other leg straight. Push yourself back into a neutral standing position, and then move into a reverse lunge with the same leg you just bent. Your knee should be just touching the floor. Return to standing and do a front kick by extending your leg out and as far up as you can.

Push-Up to Side Plank: Start in a plank position with your feet in a wide stance and your hands on the floor directly below your shoulders. Move into a push-up by bringing your chest toward the floor and pushing back up. On your way up, rotate your entire body to the right, raising your right arm and extending it toward the ceiling. Your entire body should be facing the right, with your toes rotated to face the same direction and your left arm straight. Return to center position, push up, and repeat a side plank on the left side.

The Workout

Do each movement for 30 seconds and take 10 seconds to transition to the next movement. Complete 2 rounds.

Broad Jump with 180-Degree Jump Squat Turns

Inchworm to 4 Mountain Climbers (single count)

Lateral Lunge to Reverse Lunge to Front Kicks (right on the first round, left on the second round)

Push-Up to Side Planks

Recover for 20 seconds before starting the second round.

8. 30-Minute Body-Weight Workout

I hate burpees, and every time I complain about them in class, my instructor tells me that they don't like me either. That retort is not so helpful, but there is no better full-body workout than a burpee. Not using weights in this 30-minute workout actually makes it even more challenging, as you're working with all your body weight.

Part 1

The Movements

Burpees: Begin in a standing position with your feet shoulder width apart. Lower your body into a squatting position, placing your hands on the floor in front of you. Kick your feet back so that you are in push-up position. Keep your hands firmly on the ground to support your body and drop your chest completely to the floor (this is not a push-up, which is a more controlled, smoother motion). Bring your chest back up. Jump your feet back to their original position outside of your hands, stand back up by coming back through the squat position, and complete the move by jumping into the air.

Sit-Ups: Sit with your knees bent and your feet flat on the floor. Lie on your back and put your hands behind your head. Raise yourself up so that you are sitting upright to complete one rep.

Air Squats: Stand with your feet hip width apart. Sit back as though you were sitting down on a chair, keeping your chest up. To complete the movement, stand back up and squeeze your glutes as you return to the upright position.

Box Jumps: Using a box jump or a bench, stand with your feet shoulder width apart, at a comfortable distance from the box. To initiate the movement, drop into a shallow squat, then extend your hips, swing your arms, and push your feet against the floor to propel yourself onto the box. Land quietly in a squat position and finish the movement by fully opening your hips and standing tall on top of the box. Step back down one foot at a time. You can also use a step or a secure bench that won't tip over.

The Workout

15-Minute AMRAP (as many rounds as possible): Complete the following sequence as many times as possible within the 15-minute time cap.

10 Burpees

10 Sit-Ups

10 Air Squats

10 Box Jumps

Rest for 1 minute.

Part 2

The Movements

Jumping Jacks: Do simple jumping jacks, making sure to reach your hands all the way out and above your head.

Bicycle Crunches: Sit on the floor with your knees bent and your feet flat on the floor. Lie on your back and put your hands behind your head. Raise your knees to a 45-degree angle while pressing your lower back into the floor and lifting your upper body off the floor. Begin cycling your legs, moving each knee to the opposite elbow. Continue to alternate your knees, using a fluid motion.

Walking Lunges: Start by standing tall, and then take a large step forward with your right leg into a lunge, bending both knees at a 90-degree angle, with your left knee just touching the floor. Stand up by bringing your left leg to meet your right leg, propelling your body by driving your right foot into the ground. Step forward with your left leg and repeat.

Burpee Tuck Jumps: Begin in a standing position with your feet shoulder width apart. Lower your body into a squatting position, placing your hands on the floor in front of you. Kick your feet back so that you are in push-up position. Keep your hands firmly on the ground to support your body and drop your chest to the floor (this is not a push-up, which is a more controlled, smoother motion). Bring your chest back up. Jump your feet back to their original position outside of your hands, stand back up by coming back through the squat position, and complete the move by jumping into the air, bringing your knees up and grabbing them with your arms before landing back on your feet.

The Workout

15-Minute AMRAP (as many rounds as possible): Complete the following sequence as many times as possible within the 15-minute time cap.

20 Jumping Jacks

15 Bicycle Crunches (double count; right leg then left leg = 1 bicycle crunch)

10 Walking Lunges

5 Burpee Tuck Jumps

9. 15-Minute Medicine Ball Workout

Aside from being a great stress-reliever—check out the medicine ball slam—a medicine ball is a great tool for your body because it not only requires you to bear weight but also requires you to stabilize every muscle. This workout works your shoulders and core a lot, really targeting the spare tire area—your lower belly and love handles.

Part 1

The Movements

Medicine Ball Thrusters: Holding the medicine ball with both hands at chest level, squat down with your butt back. As you rise to a standing position, press the medicine ball up to the ceiling, fully extending your arms overhead. Your legs should really provide the momentum to drive your arms up; ensure that you are pressing up your arms and standing simultaneously.

Close-Grip Push-Ups on Medicine Ball: Start in a plank position with your feet in a wide stance and your hands balancing on the medicine ball. Lower your chest toward the medicine ball while keeping your elbows in close to your sides. Push yourself back up to the starting position to complete one rep.

Reverse Lunge to Medicine Ball Twists: Start with the medicine ball in both hands at chest level and your arms extended in front of your chest. Step backwards with your right leg into a reverse lunge. At the bottom of the movement, both knees should be forming a 90-degree angle with your back knee just touching the floor. Rotate your arms and upper body to twist toward your front leg while keeping the medicine ball extended. Return to standing and repeat the exercise, stepping backwards with your left leg.

Tuck-Ups with Medicine Ball: Sit on the floor with your knees bent and your feet floating a few inches above the ground while holding the medicine ball in front of your chest. Extend the ball overhead while simultaneously extending your legs out straight. To complete the movement, tuck back into to the starting position.

The Workout

Strength Section: Do each movement for 45 seconds and rest for 15 seconds. Complete 2 rounds.

Recommended medicine ball weight: 8 to 14 pounds

Medicine Ball Thrusters

Close-Grip Push-Ups on Medicine Ball

Reverse Lunge to Medicine Ball Twists

Tuck-Ups with Medicine Ball

Part 2

The Movements

Squat Thrust to Overhead Presses: Place your hands on the medicine ball in front of you and jump your feet back into plank position. Jump your feet back to your hands, with your feet landing to the outside of the medicine ball as if you were at the bottom of a squat. Stand up with the medicine ball at your chest and then press the medicine ball overhead to complete one rep.

Medicine Ball Slams: Stand with your feet hip width apart and with the medicine ball at chest height. Reach overhead with the ball, and using all of your force, slam the ball down directly in front of you on the floor.

Russian Twists: Sit on the floor with your knees bent and your feet floating a few inches above the ground (to modify the exercise, keep your feet on the ground for balance), and lean back so your torso is at a 45-degree angle to the floor. Hold the medicine ball with both hands, and rotate your torso to one side and then to the other side. Keep your back straight and not rounded as you rotate.

The Workout

7-Minute FHIX (functional high-intensity mix): Complete as many rounds as possible in 3 minutes of the following movements. Rest for 1 minute. Then do another 3 minutes of the same movements.

6 Squat Thrust to Overhead Presses

8 Medicine Ball Slams

10 Russian Twists

Rest for 1 minute.

10. 30-Minute Rowing Workout

I'm convinced the rowing machine is trying to kill me, but according to the amazing Fhitting Room trainers, it's actually a fabulous low-impact, total-body workout. It's both aerobic and anaerobic and pushes your endurance like no other machine at the gym. I may not trust the rower, but I trust these trainers!

The Workout

Record the distance (meters) you row in the first half of the workout and try to match your meters when you go back up the ladder.

4-minute row for meters

Rest for 1 minute.

3-minute row for meters

Rest for 1 minute.

2-minute row for meters

Rest for 1 minute.

1-minute row for meters

Rest for 1 minute.

1-minute row for meters

Rest for 1 minute.

2-minute row

Rest for 1 minute.

3-minute row

Rest for 1 minute.

4-minute row

Chapter 5

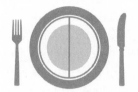

Real-Life Applications

A PLAN CAN ONLY WORK WELL if you can take it everywhere with you. It's certainly easier to follow a healthy meal plan when you're preparing all your own food at home, but that's not realistic for most people. Here are some tips and guidelines for how to take the Diet Detox out of the house and into the real world with you.

Social Scene

One of the biggest concerns that both my clients and my friends share with me is that they don't want to "be that person" at the dinner table. By "that person," they mean the person who asks questions in restaurants, the one who orders a different side with a dish, the one who gets the dressing on the side, or even worse, the one who doesn't have a drink.

If you want to lose weight or feel better, then you are going to have to change the way you eat. Period. This includes meals in social situations. Since you are reading this book, chances are you are a grown adult. Being an adult means being able to say no to peer pressure and making your own decisions based on what's best for you.

When we dine out at restaurants or even at someone's home, we lose a little bit of control over what goes into our food. You can be like Meg Ryan in *When Harry Met Sally* and ask a hundred questions (it's not a bad thing), or you can simply do your best and ask for sauces or dressings on the side, which can be loaded with secret sugars.

What's most important when it comes to dining out, especially if it's something that you do frequently, is that you need to flip that switch in your brain telling you that it's a once-in-a-lifetime opportunity. I have one client in particular, a very successful gentleman who had been struggling with his weight for years before coming to see me. Anytime he travels or almost anytime he dines out, he gets pizza. Whenever I question him about it, he says, "Well, this place is known for its pizza, so I had to have some." Every. Single. Time. So I finally had to call him out on it, much to his displeasure. Every single restaurant that he goes to can't be famous for its pizza. Plus, I see his food diaries and I know the restaurants he's eating at, so I am even more confident that pizza is not their specialty. I was finally able to get through to him when I spoke to him very clearly. We talked about intentional indulgences. If you're going to indulge, it better be worth it and planned for. I told him, "Listen, you have been to fabulous pizza places and you will be at many more. Don't waste your pizza on the mediocre stuff." That clicked for him. The takeaway here is that not every meal out is an occasion. If you have planned for your intentional indulgence, then great, enjoy every bite without guilt. Remember, it's guilt that leads us to weight gain. When we feel guilty about our food choice, we eat more of that food and enjoy it less, and all of this causes us to make another bad decision.

I also have clients who feel awkward not drinking when they are at social events. One client in particular said she was worried about making her companions feel uncomfortable; she feared that if she didn't order a drink, they would feel guilty about drinking or might not order a drink. It wasn't obvious to her that she wasn't the one with the issue here. If her friends or acquaintances couldn't be around her if she didn't have a drink, then that was their problem, not hers. And their issues shouldn't get in the way of the goals she has for her health and body. If you can't be comfortable ordering a club soda with lime at a bar, then you shouldn't be at that bar in the first place.

The lesson here is that you can't let other people's issues mess up the way you want to eat or drink. You shouldn't judge them for their choices, and they shouldn't judge you for yours. If they do, I'm going to have to suggest finding some new friends.

Q. Please don't tell me to stop drinking if I want to lose weight—anyone who says that deserves to be unfriended on Facebook.

A. Here's the deal. You don't need to stop drinking to lose weight, but it will happen more quickly if you're willing to dry out for a bit. That said, if you want to lose weight and still drink alcohol, you need to drink smarter than you would normally. There are two rules that work for this, depending on your drinking habits and your social style. The first works best for people who need to socialize for work events and have a hard time just getting sparkling water, while the second works best for people with an all-or-nothing attitude to alcohol.

Boozy Rule #1

If you need to drink socially for work and feel uncomfortable sipping nonalcoholic options—or just don't want to—set the maximum number of drinks you can have for an entire week. This number varies widely for my clients, but the maximum I give per week is six. Then each night out you can have some drinks, so long as you don't go over that limit for the week.

Boozy Rule #2

Pick two nights (or days if you're into that) a week that you drink. The rest of the time you are totally dry. The only qualification to this rule is that you can never have more than three drinks per night. Too much booze equals poor food choices. It's a simple math equation!

Restaurant Rules

1. Plan ahead. It's great to read the menu ahead of time online. This way, you will know what you are going to eat and won't be swayed when the other diners at the table try to get the blooming onion for you to share.

2. Speaking of sharing, it doesn't work. Most of the time, sharing leads to poor choices or unintentional indulgences. Just because you and your friends "split a dessert" doesn't mean it doesn't count as eating dessert. If you want to share something, be in charge of ordering it and make sure you count it toward your indulgence or starch if it falls into those categories.

3. No freebies. This includes anything the server brings to the table that you didn't specifically order, such as bread, chips, or cookies. If you didn't order it, you shouldn't eat it.

4. No drinks until the food arrives. I'm pro-booze when appropriate, but drinking before your meal arrives sets you up to fail. Either you drink more because you finish your drink before your food is done or you reach for those freebies while you sip your drink because alcohol inhibits good decision-making and can amplify your body's hunger cues.

5. One dish must be mainly veggies. If you're having more than one course, then one of them needs to be veggie heavy—and fries do not count. It's easy to get a side of green veggies at most places.

6. If you are struggling with concerns about sticking out when you order, order last. By the time the server gets to you, everyone else is usually back into the conversation and couldn't care less about what you eat.

Q. Is it better to get olive oil with the breadbasket instead of butter?

A. First of all, *step away from the breadbasket*. You're missing the big picture here: most of the time you shouldn't be eating the contents of the breadbasket at all.

While a few establishments may have breadbaskets worthy of an intentional indulgence, the majority of the breads served in restaurants are loaded with white flour and are somewhat stale. Also, we tend to eat bread in addition to what we order at a restaurant, not in place of something else. So at the end of the meal, we've added extra calories and sugar for something that's not even that tasty.

Traveling and Traipsing

The fear of traveling while dieting is strong for some people. But travel is also a great excuse to overindulge for many others! Many of my clients travel a lot, for business and for pleasure, and while it's a little trickier to stay healthy on the road, it's certainly doable. I set some different rules for traveling, depending on whether it's for business or pleasure. As tough as I am on my clients and you, the reader, I also get that we all need a chance to chill out.

If you are following the Diet Detox correctly, you shouldn't be feeling deprived, which should already help set you up for success when you travel—unlike people who starve themselves before a vacation to get bikini ready and then down every frozen drink, ice cream cone, or anything else in sight once they're there. I can't tell you how many women come to me after their honeymoons because they gained weight while they were away.

So how do we travel without ruining all our hard work? If possible, try to avoid traveling for the first week or two of the Diet Detox, while you learn the plan. Then when you travel, follow these three steps:

1. Always be prepared! This is when taking a few minutes to pack a snack makes a huge difference. Bars (snack ones, not booze ones) are a lifesaver here. See page 196 for brands I recommend.
2. Choose your poison. If you want to eat French fries on the beach or drink a frozen drink or two daily, then you need to give something else up. I often tell my clients to limit their starches to one serving or none to make room for the extra indulgences.
3. Don't mess with breakfast. Whether you're on vacation or traveling for work, breakfast is often the one meal at which you have the most control. Beef up (pun intended) the protein and the fiber here. Nothing beats an omelet loaded with veggies. Stay away from the continental breakfast—muffins and pastries are dessert!

It's also important to remember that it's OK for you to be watching what you eat. There's nothing wrong with being in a meeting and taking off half the bread on your sandwich or ordering a salad—it's important that you make yourself a priority when it comes to your food choices whenever possible. Maybe you'll even motivate your colleagues to do the same. It's the same deal with drinking when you're out (see "Social Scene" on page 117); if you are not drinking and your healthy choice

Q. Seriously, is it possible to go on vacation and not gain weight? I have yet to have that happen.

A. This is a constant struggle for a lot of my clients, and I will tell you what I tell them for a fraction of the cost (the price of this book): you need to make a choice while you are on vacation, a decision about where you're going to define boundaries. This is the only time I recommend having very clear-cut guidelines, but it's for a short period of time. So if you want to drink when you are on vacation, then choose to avoid all starches instead. If you want to indulge in starches, then avoid booze and dessert. It is a trade-off, but it works. It is also smart to start each day of your vacation with a protein-heavy breakfast, as it can set the tone for the rest of the day. But the best method is to pick your metaphorical poison and ignore all others.

makes other people uncomfortable, that's their issue, not yours. If you want that bread, drink, or whatever, then eat it, but there is no reason to be forced to eat a mediocre sandwich just because you're at a work meeting.

Case Study: Jess

Jess is a mom of two young children, ages three and one. When she came to me, she told me that she hadn't lost the baby weight fully from her first son before she got pregnant with her daughter and now, a year later, she saw no hope of ever losing the weight. When we went over her typical day, I saw that Jess didn't eat actual grown-up meals. She ate scraps of her kids' food or random leftovers. She didn't get enough sleep and hadn't exercised since before her first pregnancy. I really had my work cut out for me here.

I first addressed the food issue. We weren't even ready to get to Rule #1 about protein and fiber because Jess first had to just make some food for herself. She had been sharing her son's waffles and bagels and her daughter's leftover yogurt for breakfast most days, or some variation of that. I looked her in the eye and actually said, "Jess, you deserve better than your kids' leftovers in the morning." I think that hit close to home, but the idea of making another breakfast was overwhelming.

We went over the rules and worked out how to apply them to her daily life. I added an 11th one for her: "Don't eat the kids' leftovers." Since breakfast was the most hectic, we came up with a few easy additions to her morning that wouldn't overwhelm her. The first was a smoothie that she and the kids could eat. She'd make it with greens, Greek yogurt, and a small amount of fruit, then pour some into a glass for herself with some chia seeds. Then she'd add some extra fruit and a bit of honey and blend more of the smoothie for her kids. This was one dish that all three of them could enjoy, and now Jess was getting the nutrition she needed while not throwing off her day by eating sweet starches in the morning. Other options we came up with were hard-boiled eggs and an apple with nut butter. The kids liked these choices too.

Once Jess learned that the rules of the Diet Detox were not going to take up a huge amount of time and that this wasn't a plan to start and stop, she slowly got the hang of it. We came up with great easy meal options for her and her kids, plus snacks to keep in her diaper bag that weren't Goldfish, so she always had a healthy option around. It was amazing that she always left the house with a snack and water for her kids but never thought to do the same for herself. I told her that if I could get her to take care of herself half as well as she was taking care of her kids, then we would have a very easy time.

In our next session, Jess was laughing because between her meals and her snacks, it felt like she was always eating. While she wasn't able to make time for the gym yet, she started putting her youngest in the stroller for one of her naps and used that time to do a fast-paced walk a couple of times per week. She saved her intentional indulgence for the weekends to have a piece of cake or a slice of pizza at the never-ending birthday parties they'd attend regularly. She was also sleeping better, thanks to her new supplement regime plus her extra exercise. After six months, Jess had lost 27 pounds and was back to her pre-pregnancy weight. She's not eating leftover grilled cheese crust anymore and is finally putting herself on her list of priorities.

Mom Life

My mom clients are often the most interesting to work with as I relate to them on such a personal level. Plenty of dads also fit into this category, but it's usually the moms I see in my practice. They are devoted and caring and often sacrifice their own needs in favor of their kids'. So when a mom doesn't understand why she can't lose weight, it's often because she doesn't put her own needs anywhere on her daily priority list. Healthy eating and exercise come after everything else.

This is where I can relate all too well. I'm a mom of two amazing girls, plus I run a business. Finding time for myself is sometimes impossible, and it always feels like something needs to give. Fitting in some "me time" means either I work less or I see less of my kids. Whichever route I go, I always feel guilty. It wasn't until my eldest was in preschool that I was able to really devote time to my own needs. When this happened, it was quite an awakening. Exercising, or merely sitting down and having lunch without the computer or someone who needs a sippy cup, actually made me better at the other things I was doing. Suddenly work felt less like a chore, and I was much more present when I was with my daughter.

This is the advice I always give to my mom clients: if you take care of yourself and make doing that a priority—maybe not the top priority but at least somewhere on the list—you will be better at taking care of other people too.

Case Study: George

George's job requires him to be on the road about three days a week. When he came to me, his weight was creeping up to 300 pounds and the long car trips were taking a physical toll on his body. Since his body was hurting so much during the trips, he would often stay in the car and use a fast-food drive-through instead of getting out and feeling how stiff and sore he was. Changing his travel schedule was not a possibility, but we were able to make some changes that made a pretty big impact. Every Sunday, I had him make a bag for a week's worth of healthy snacks he could take on the road. I gave him a list of foods to order in bulk, including nuts, grass-fed jerky, and bars. Plus, I had him stock up on apples or other fruit he could cut up and bring along. All this protein and fiber would hold him over until he got to his destination.

Sometimes just being prepared is the best thing you can do to set yourself up for success. I couldn't believe that this very bright guy didn't think of packing himself healthy snacks, and when I asked him why, he said he always forgot to and would just grab something on the road to make it easier. We had a tough-love conversation about this, as grabbing fast food didn't make his life any easier. A snowstorm in which you are stranded with no other options is one thing (that happened to me with my kids!), but a planned road trip that you take three times a week is a totally different story.

The other rule I gave him was that he had to take a break every 90 minutes to move his body. This was a big one since he was typically in his car for up to 3 hours at a stretch, six times a week. As I mentioned earlier, nothing brings awareness to your body like *moving* it, so simply stopping to use the bathroom or fill the car up with gas gave him an opportunity to move. I also encouraged him to buy a pedometer or to use his smartphone to count his steps. Since those travel days were so inactive, it was good to have a goal of how much to move. For him, regular days were 10,000 steps and travel days were 5,000, a realistic goal but still a bit of a challenge. Once we added these simple elements, the transformation was amazing. This man had been steadily gaining 10 to 15 pounds a year, and now he was losing about 2 pounds a week. Major success!

Chapter 6

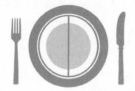

Diet Plan Review

H ERE'S THE PLAN mapped out for you all in one place, including the one-week Kick-Starter, the Diet Detox rules, a day in the life on the Diet Detox, and two weeks of living the Diet Detox. For a printable version of the rules as well as a blank copy of the food diary, visit my website, b-nutritious.com.

Protein (P): Animal products, dairy products, nuts, seeds, beans

Fiber (F): Fruits, vegetables

Starch (S): Grains, bread, quinoa, sweet potato, butternut squash

One-Week Kick-Starter

1. Every morning before breakfast, take 1 scoop (14.8 grams) FibeHER fiber supplement with an 8-ounce glass of water.
2. Every meal needs to have a serving of protein and a serving of fiber (P & F). Each snack should include protein and/or fiber. You can pick one of the three options from the protein category and one of the fiber options (see the meal guidelines on page 13). If you are still hungry, you may have an additional fiber.

3. Add fat to your protein or fiber in every meal. Cook your eggs in grass-fed butter or coconut oil. Use olive oil on your salad or sauté your vegetables in ghee. Add half of an avocado to any meal. Note: Dairy and nut products already contain fat, so they'll do double duty as fat and protein. If you have a full-fat Greek yogurt for breakfast, then you don't have to think about fat—it's already included.

4. You are allotted only one serving of starch (S) per day. Choose one of the three options on page 13 at lunch or at dinner. I recommend saving your starch for lunch or dinner to keep your blood sugar levels even and help you sleep better.

5. Try to follow the serving sizes I recommend on page 17, but do not go hungry! Remember, this isn't about deprivation; it's about getting back on track. If you're truly hungry and you're not just bored or thirsty, add more of the protein or fiber options to your meal or snack. But before you do, read "Are You Truly Hungry?" on page 10.

6. No alcohol. It's one week—don't complain.

7. Drink a minimum of around 2 liters or 64 ounces of water a day. Add lemon or lime for flavor. Unsweetened tea is also fine, as is coffee, but limit it to 2 cups a day with ¼ cup of milk or a nondairy alternative. No sugar, please!

8. Aim to drink 1 to 2 cups of dandelion root tea per day (see page 197). Dandelion is a lot more than a weed. Tea made from its roots can boost weight loss, improve digestion, and regulate blood sugar levels, which makes it the perfect addition to this one-week program and to your diet afterwards. It's also caffeine-free, so feel free to drink it any time of day. My favorite brand is Alvita, which is both organic and high quality.

9. Need something sweet? You can have 1 ounce of good-quality dark chocolate a day. For the Kick-Starter program it must be at least 80 percent cocoa.

Meal Guidelines (see page 17 for serving sizes)

Pre-breakfast

FibeHER fiber supplement

Breakfast

Protein *(pick one):* Eggs, full-fat yogurt, nut butter

Fiber *(pick one):* Berries, spinach, apple

Lunch

Protein *(pick one):* Sliced turkey, canned/jarred tuna, chicken

Fiber *(pick one):* Mixed greens, cucumbers, peppers

Starch *(pick one):* Multigrain bread, rice, whole-wheat wrap

Add a fat (see below)

Snack

Protein *(pick one):* Nuts, full-fat yogurt, hummus

Fiber *(pick one):* Berries, carrots, apple

Dinner

Protein *(pick one):* Fish, chicken, beef

Fiber *(pick one):* Mixed greens, cauliflower, broccoli

Starch *(if you didn't eat a starch at lunch, pick one):* Rice, quinoa, sweet potato

Add a fat (see below)

Suggested Fats to Be Used in Every Meal

Olive oil, coconut oil, avocado, guacamole, butter (ideally grass-fed), ghee. Note that full-fat yogurt, nut butters, eggs, and nuts also count as fats.

Condiments and Seasonings

Salt, pepper, mustard (no sugar added), balsamic vinegar, lemon, lime, tomato sauce (no sugar added), salsa (no sugar added), onions, garlic, herbs and spices, tamari

The Diet Detox

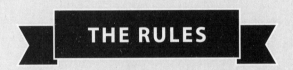

THE RULES

1. Eat protein and fiber at every meal.
2. Check your starch.
3. Clock your meals.
4. Eat fat.
5. Watch the sugar.
6. Indulge intentionally.
7. Supplement smartly.
8. Get some sleep.
9. Drink water.
10. Exercise.

A Day in the Life of the Diet Detox

Breakfast: P & F

Snack: P &/or F

Lunch: P & F + S

Snack: P &/or F

Dinner: P & F + S + end 12 to 14 hours before your next meal

Plus: Supplements, exercise, sleeping, and drinking water

Two Weeks on the Diet Detox

Here is a two-week eating plan on the Diet Detox. I've utilized some of the recipes found on page 143 to show you where they fit into your day. Use this as a resource as you transition out of the one-week Kick-Starter.

MONDAY		
Breakfast		**Time: 7:30 AM**
2 Broccoli and Cheddar Egg Muffins*		ⓟ ⓕ S
		P F S
		P F S
Snack		**Time: 11:00 AM**
Apple		
Almonds		
Lunch		**Time: 1:30 PM**
½ turkey sandwich		ⓟ F Ⓢ
Small vegetable soup		P ⓕ S
		P F S
		P F S
Snack		**Time: 3:30 PM**
Mint chocolate Health Warrior Chia Bar		
Dinner		**Time: 7:00 PM**
Poached and Shredded Chicken*		ⓟ F S
Sautéed broccoli		P ⓕ S
Rice		P F Ⓢ
1 ounce dark chocolate		P F S
Other		
Water: 2 liters		
Exercise: Walking		
Supplements: FibeHER, Ultimate Omega 2X Mini, Nightly One, Beautiflora		

*See recipe section.

TUESDAY		
Breakfast		*Time:* **7:00** AM
Yogurt		Ⓟ F S
½ cup berries		P Ⓕ S
		P F S
Snack		*Time:* **10:00** AM
Mini Perfect Bar		
Lunch		*Time:* **1:00** PM
Almond butter and sliced banana sandwich		Ⓟ Ⓕ Ⓢ
Sliced red peppers		P Ⓕ S
		P F S
		P F S
Snack		*Time:* **3:30** PM
Orange		
1 ounce dark chocolate		
Dinner		*Time:* **7:00** PM
Mom's Wild Salmon*		Ⓟ F S
Roasted cauliflower and broccoli		P Ⓕ S
		P F S
		P F S
Other		
Water: 2 liters		
Exercise: Four 15-minute walks throughout the day		
Supplements: FibeHER, Ultimate Omega 2X Mini, Nightly One, Beautiflora		

*See recipe section.

Breakfast	Time: 7:00 AM
2 pieces chicken-apple breakfast sausage	Ⓟ F S
½ grapefruit	P Ⓕ S
	P F S

Snack	Time:

Lunch	Time: 11:30 AM
Summer Salad* with a scoop of tuna salad	Ⓟ Ⓕ S
1 ounce dark chocolate	P F S
	P F S
	P F S

Snack	Time: 3:00 PM
Birthday cupcake (intentional indulgence)	

Dinner	Time: 6:30 PM
Orange-Glazed Lamb Chops*	Ⓟ F S
Mixed salad	P Ⓕ S
	P F S
	P F S

Other
Water: 2 liters
Exercise: Yoga DVD
Supplements: FibeHER, Ultimate Omega 2X Mini, Nightly One, Beautiflora

WEDNESDAY

*See recipe section.

THURSDAY		
Breakfast		*Time:* 6:30 AM
Melon bowl		P Ⓕ S
Cottage cheese		Ⓟ F S
		P F S
Snack		*Time:* 10:15 AM
Pistachios		
Lunch		*Time:* 12:45 PM
Turkey sandwich with a lettuce wrap		Ⓟ Ⓕ S
Sliced cucumbers with vinegar		P Ⓕ S
		P F S
		P F S
Snack		*Time:* 4:00 PM
Grapes		
1 ounce cheese		
Dinner		*Time:* 7:00 PM
Chili-Lime Chicken Strips*		Ⓟ F S
Coconutty Quinoa*		P F Ⓢ
Broccoli		P Ⓕ S
		P F S
Other		
Water: 2 liters		
Exercise: None		
Supplements: FibeHER, Ultimate Omega 2X Mini, Nightly One, Beautiflora		

*See recipe section.

Breakfast			**Time:** 8:30 AM	
Poached eggs over sautéed kale	Ⓟ	Ⓕ	S
	P	F	S
	P	F	S

Snack			**Time:**	

Lunch			**Time:** 12:30 PM	
Burger with no bun, over salad	Ⓟ	Ⓕ	S
	P	F	S
	P	F	S
	P	F	S

Snack			**Time:** 3:45 PM	
Yogurt with ¼ cup approved granola			

Dinner			**Time:** 7:00 PM	
Steamed Cod with Ginger and Scallions*	Ⓟ	F	S
Cold Soba Noodles*	P	F	Ⓢ
Small salad	P	Ⓕ	S
	P	F	S

Other
Water: 2 liters
Exercise: 35 minutes HIIT
Supplements: FibeHER, Ultimate Omega 2X Mini, Nightly One, Beautiflora

FRIDAY

*See recipe section.

Breakfast			*Time:* 8:00 AM
Sliced smoked salmon with capers	Ⓟ	F	S
½ avocado	P	F	S
1 pear	P	Ⓕ	S
Snack			*Time:* 11:00 AM
Small fruit salad topped with chia seeds			
Lunch			*Time:* 1:30 PM
Caesar salad with chicken, with no croutons	Ⓟ	Ⓕ	S
	P	F	S
	P	F	S
	P	F	S
Snack			*Time:* 4:00 PM
Kale chips			
Dinner			*Time:* 7:30 PM
Greek salad	P	Ⓕ	S
Beef kebabs	Ⓟ	F	S
	P	F	S
	P	F	S
Other			
Water: 2 liters			
Exercise: 45 minutes cardio plus light weights			
Supplements: FibeHER, Ultimate Omega 2X Mini, Nightly One, Beautiflora			

SATURDAY

*See recipe section.

Breakfast			Time: 8:30 AM
Pancakes (intentional indulgence)	P F S		Ⓘ
	P F S		
	P F S		

Snack	Time:

Lunch		Time: 1:00 PM
Large mixed green salad with grilled shrimp	Ⓟ Ⓕ S	
	P F S	
	P F S	
	P F S	

Snack	Time: 3:30 PM
Sliced red peppers	

Dinner		Time: 6:00 PM
Turkey Lettuce Tacos*	Ⓟ Ⓕ S	
Roasted Peppers and Onions*	P Ⓕ S	
Guacamole	P F S	
	P F S	

Other
Water: 2 liters
Exercise: 1 hour walking around the city
Supplements: FibeHER, Ultimate Omega 2X Mini, Nightly One, Beautiflora

SUNDAY

*See recipe section.

MONDAY		
Breakfast		**Time:** 6:30 AM
2 hard-boiled eggs		(P) F S
Apple		P (F) S
		P F S
Snack		**Time:** 9:30 AM
Yogurt		
Chia seeds		
Lunch		**Time:** 12:30 PM
Chicken		(P) F S
Broccoli		P (F) S
Sweet potato		P F (S)
1 ounce dark chocolate		P F S
Snack		**Time:** 3:00 PM
10 Mary's Gone Crackers		
Hummus		
Dinner		**Time:** 6:45 PM
Sautéed shrimp		(P) F S
Cauliflower Tumeric Rice*		P (F) S
		P F S
		P F S
Other		
Water: 2 liters		
Exercise: 30 Minutes HIIT		
Supplements: FibeHER, Ultimate Omega 2X Mini, Nightly One, Beautiflora		

*See recipe section.

TUESDAY	**Breakfast**	*Time:* **7:00** AM
	Yogurt	Ⓟ F S
	½ cup berries	P Ⓕ S
		P F S
	Snack	*Time:* **10:00** AM
	Mini Perfect Bar	
	Lunch	*Time:* **1:30** PM
	Almond butter and sliced banana sandwich	Ⓟ Ⓕ Ⓢ
	Sliced red peppers	P Ⓕ S
		P F S
		P F S
	Snack	*Time:* **3:30** PM
	Orange	
	1 ounce dark chocolate	
	Dinner	*Time:* **7:00** PM
	Mom's Wild Salmon*	Ⓟ F S
	Roasted cauliflower and broccoli	P Ⓕ S
		P F S
		P F S
	Other	
	Water: 2 liters	
	Exercise: Four 15-minute walks throughout the day	
	Supplements: FibeHER, Ultimate Omega 2X Mini, Nightly One, Beautiflora	

*See recipe section.

WEDNESDAY	Breakfast	Time: 7:00 AM
	2 pieces chicken-apple breakfast sausage	(P) F S
	½ grapefruit	P (F) S
		P F S
	Snack	**Time:**
	Lunch	**Time: 11:30 AM**
	Summer Salad* with a scoop of tuna salad	(P) (F) S
	1 ounce dark chocolate	P F S
		P F S
		P F S
	Snack	**Time: 3:00 PM**
	Birthday cupcake (intentional indulgence)	
	Dinner	**Time: 6:30 PM**
	Orange-Glazed Lamb Chops*	(P) F S
	Mixed salad	P (F) S
		P F S
		P F S
	Other	
	Water: 2 liters	
	Exercise: Yoga DVD	
	Supplements: FibeHER, Ultimate Omega 2X Mini, Nightly One, Beautiflora	

*See recipe section.

THURSDAY		
Breakfast		*Time:* 6:30 AM
Melon bowl		P Ⓕ S
Cottage cheese		Ⓟ F S
		P F S
Snack		*Time:* 10:15 AM
Pistachios		
Lunch		*Time:* 12:45 PM
Turkey sandwich with a lettuce wrap		Ⓟ Ⓕ S
Sliced cucumbers with vinegar		P Ⓕ S
		P F S
		P F S
Snack		*Time:* 4:00 PM
Grapes		
1 ounce cheese		
Dinner		*Time:* 7:00 PM
Chili-Lime Chicken Strips*		Ⓟ F S
Coconutty Quinoa*		P F Ⓢ
Broccoli		P Ⓕ S
		P F S
Other		
Water: 2 liters		
Exercise: None		
Supplements: FibeHER, Ultimate Omega 2X Mini, Nightly One, Beautiflora		

*See recipe section.

FRIDAY	**Breakfast**		**Time:** 8:30 AM
	Poached eggs over sautéed kale		Ⓟ Ⓕ S
			P F S
			P F S
	Snack		**Time:**
	Lunch		**Time:** 12:30 PM
	Burger with no bun, over salad		Ⓟ Ⓕ S
			P F S
			P F S
			P F S
	Snack		**Time:** 3:45 PM
	Yogurt with ¼ cup approved granola		
	Dinner		**Time:** 7:00 PM
	Steamed Cod with Ginger and Scallions*		Ⓟ F S
	Cold Soba Noodles*		P F Ⓢ
	Small salad		P Ⓕ S
			P F S
	Other		
	Water: 2 liters		
	Exercise: 35 Minutes HIIT		
	Supplements: FibeHER, Ultimate Omega 2X Mini, Nightly One, Beautiflora		

*See recipe section.

SATURDAY	**Breakfast**	*Time:* 8:00 AM
	Sliced smoked salmon with capers	Ⓟ F S
	½ avocado	P F S
	1 pear	P Ⓕ S
	Snack	*Time:* 11:00 AM
	Small fruit salad topped with chia seeds	
	Lunch	*Time:* 1:30 PM
	Caesar salad with chicken, with no croutons	Ⓟ Ⓕ S
		P F S
		P F S
		P F S
	Snack	*Time:* 4:00 PM
	Kale chips	
	Dinner	*Time:* 6:45 PM
	Greek salad	P Ⓕ S
	Beef kebabs	Ⓟ F S
		P F S
		P F S
	Other	
	Water: 2 liters	
	Exercise: 45 minutes cardio plus light weights	
	Supplements: FibeHER, Ultimate Omega 2X Mini, Nightly One, Beautiflora	

*See recipe section.

SUNDAY	**Breakfast**	***Time:* 8:30 AM**
	Pancakes (intentional indulgence)	P F S
		P F S
		P F S
	Snack	***Time:***
	Lunch	***Time:* 1:00 PM**
	Large mixed green salad with grilled shrimp	Ⓟ Ⓕ S
		P F S
		P F S
		P F S
	Snack	***Time:* 3:30 PM**
	Sliced red peppers	
	Dinner	***Time:* 6:00 PM**
	Turkey Lettuce Tacos*	Ⓟ Ⓕ S
	Roasted Peppers and Onions*	P Ⓕ S
	Guacamole	P F S
		P F S
	Other	
	Water: 2 liters	
	Exercise: 1 hour walking around the city	
	Supplements: FibeHER, Ultimate Omega 2X Mini, Nightly One, Beautiflora	

*See recipe section.

Recipes

ONE CONCERN THAT CLIENTS OFTEN HAVE when they come to see me is that they're going to have to start cooking. While you don't *have* to cook, the truth is that you should whenever possible. Cooking your own food allows you to have full control over everything you eat, plus it connects you more with the food you eat. Cooking even just a few times a week can help you gain more awareness about portion sizes and can teach you to better "eyeball" how much you're eating when you're not in a controlled environment. I get that time is limited and that not everyone loves to be in the kitchen all day, so I created some recipes for simple, quick meals.

I'm not a chef. In fact, I'm far from it. But I can follow a recipe. And if I can follow a recipe, then you can too. That's all you need to do here. All the recipes have five ingredients or fewer (not including salt and pepper, cooking oil, or a garnish) and make creating your ideal plate (protein, fiber, starch) very easy. I've even organized the recipes by protein, fiber, and starch categories so all you need to do is mix and match. I've also included a section after the recipes that shows you how to build your meals and what pairs best with what.

PROTEIN

Asian-Inspired Grilled Chicken

Chicken is a great protein option, but it certainly gets boring. Not this dish! The bright flavors will pull you out of your chicken rut. Don't get stuck in the habit of always using chicken breasts; chicken thighs are just as healthy and taste much better.

Serves: 4

Ingredients

- 4 tablespoons tomato paste
- 2 tablespoons toasted sesame oil
- 3 tablespoons tamari (gluten-free soy sauce)
- 2 tablespoons sesame seeds
- 8 bone-in, skin-on chicken thighs

Directions

1. In a mixing bowl, combine the tomato paste, sesame oil, tamari, and sesame seeds and mix with a fork until incorporated.
2. Add the chicken thighs and coat well. Let them marinate in the refrigerator for at least 1 hour or overnight.
3. Preheat the oven to 375°F. Line a baking sheet with parchment paper or aluminum foil.
4. Place the chicken thighs skin side up on the lined baking sheet and bake for 35 to 40 minutes, or until fully cooked through.
5. Serve immediately.

Serve with: *Sautéed Bok Choy* (page 160) and *Fresh Quinoa Salad* (page 178)

Chili-Lime Chicken Strips

When you're focusing on protein and fiber all the time, you tend to eat a lot of chicken. To keep it from getting boring and repetitive, I like to experiment with different options and flavors. This one is a hit whether it's served warm or cold. Plate it with the Roasted Brussels Sprouts and the Fresh Quinoa Salad and it's anything but boring.

Serves: 4

Ingredients

- ⅛ teaspoon chili powder
- ½ teaspoon garlic powder
- ¼ teaspoon onion powder
- ¼ teaspoon salt
- ¼ cup fresh lime juice (about 2 limes)
- 1 pound boneless, skinless chicken breasts
- 1 tablespoon coconut oil

Directions

1. In a small bowl, mix the chili, garlic powder, onion powder, and salt.
2. Mix in the lime juice.
3. Place the lime and spice mix and the chicken in a large ziplock bag. Allow the chicken to marinate in the refrigerator for at least 1 hour.
4. Heat the coconut oil in a grill pan over medium-high heat.
5. Grill the chicken for 3 to 5 minutes on each side.
6. Let the chicken sit for about 3 minutes to let the moisture reabsorb.
7. Slice the chicken into 1-inch strips.

Serve with: *Roasted Brussels Sprouts* (page 161) and *Fresh Quinoa Salad* (page 178)

Poached and Shredded Chicken

This recipe is very useful, especially if you have your act together enough to do some meal prep on a Sunday. Poaching the chicken prevents it from drying out, and the simple flavors make this chicken perfect as an easy protein addition to any fiber choice.

Serves: 4

Ingredients

- 1 pound boneless, skinless chicken breasts
- ½ white onion, peeled and quartered
- 2 garlic cloves, crushed
- 1 tablespoon olive oil
- Kosher salt and freshly ground black pepper, to taste

Directions

1. Combine the chicken, onion, and garlic in a large saucepan. Add enough water to cover.
2. Bring to a boil and skim off any foam that bubbles to the surface.
3. Cook for 20 to 30 minutes, or until the center of the chicken is no longer pink.
4. Drain the water and discard. Place the chicken in a large bowl and set aside to cool.
5. Shred the chicken into small, thin strips.
6. Season the shredded chicken with the olive oil, salt, and pepper. Store in the fridge for up to 3 days.

Serve with: *Creamy Kale Salad* (page 169)

Turmeric-Almond Chicken Fingers

This is a healthy take on a classic kid-friendly dish.

Serves: 4

Ingredients

- 1 egg
- 1 cup almond meal
- 1 teaspoon turmeric powder
- ½ teaspoon garlic powder
- ½ teaspoon black pepper
- ½ teaspoon salt
- 1 pound boneless, skinless chicken breasts, cut into strips

Directions

1. Preheat the oven to 425°F. Line a baking sheet with parchment paper or aluminum foil.
2. In a shallow dish, beat the egg.
3. Place the almond meal, turmeric, garlic, pepper, and salt in a small bowl. Stir to combine.
4. One by one, dredge each chicken strip in the egg, wiping off any excess, then dip each into the almond meal mixture until completely coated.
5. Place the coated tenders on the lined baking sheet and bake for 20 minutes, flipping halfway through, until the outside is golden brown.

Serve with: *Cumin-Cinnamon Roasted Carrots* (page 162)

Pesto Turkey Burger

I love the extra flavor that something as simple as pesto can add to a turkey burger. It gives a bland burger a powerful flavor punch.

Serves: 4

Ingredients

- 1 pound ground turkey breast
- 1 medium onion, finely chopped
- 3 tablespoons basil pesto (homemade or store-bought)
- 2 garlic cloves, minced
- 1½ teaspoons salt
- ½ teaspoon black pepper
- 1 tablespoon coconut oil

Directions

1. In a large bowl, mix together the ground turkey, onion, pesto, garlic, salt, and pepper until evenly blended.
2. Divide the mixture into 4 equal portions and roll them into balls between your palms.
3. Flatten the balls into ½-inch-thick patties.
4. Preheat an outdoor grill or heat a greased grill pan over medium-high heat.
5. Cook the patties on each side until cooked all the way through, 4 to 5 minutes per side or until internally 165 degrees on a meat thermometer.

Serve with: *Brooke's Favorite Salad* (page 168) and *Tahini Brown Rice* (page 175)

Turkey Lettuce Tacos

This dish is simple yet seems like a more complex meal. Ground meat bundled up in a lettuce wrap is just as satisfying as a regular taco. When paired with the Roasted Peppers and Onions, it's even more filling and takes on their fajita-style flavors.

Serves: 4

Ingredients

- 1 head lettuce
- 1 teaspoon coconut oil
- 1 medium onion, finely chopped
- 1 pound ground turkey breast or ground beef (grass-fed)
- ½ teaspoon salt
- 2 avocados, pitted and sliced
- 1 cup salsa (no sugar added)

Directions

1. Trim the stem end of the lettuce so the leaves come apart. Wash and dry the leaves thoroughly and set them aside.
2. Heat the coconut oil in a large pan over medium-high heat. Add the onion and cook until translucent, about 5 minutes.
3. Add the ground turkey or beef to the pan and cook for about 3 minutes, using a spoon to break up the larger clumps.
4. Sprinkle in the salt, stir, and continue cooking until almost all the liquid in the pan has evaporated, about 2 more minutes.
5. Remove from the heat and transfer the turkey to a bowl to cool.
6. To assemble, use a large spoon to scoop the turkey into the lettuce leaves. Add the avocados and top with the salsa.

Serve with: *Roasted Peppers and Onions* (page 165)

Spiced Beef Burger

Burgers are an easy option and I love mixing the beef with whatever spices I grab from my spice rack. These particular spices are far from exotic, but they make a plain burger so much more satisfying.

Serves: 4

Ingredients

- 1 pound ground beef (grass-fed)
- 2 garlic cloves, minced
- ½ teaspoon ground cumin
- ½ teaspoon paprika
- ½ teaspoon salt
- ½ teaspoon black pepper

Directions

1. Preheat an outdoor grill or heat a grill pan over medium heat.
2. Add the ground beef to a large bowl and combine with the garlic, cumin, paprika, salt, and pepper.
3. Shape the mixture into 4 round patties (if you prefer, you can make 6 to 8 smaller patties).
4. Place the patties on the grill or grill pan, pressing them down to flatten them.
5. Cook the patties until browned, about 4 minutes per side for medium rare, or 5 to 6 minutes per side for medium.

Serve with: *Sweet Potato Wedges* (page 186)

Orange-Glazed Lamb Chops

I love the brightness that the orange zest gives to this dish. In my house, my kids call these "lamb chop lollipops"—it's certainly fun to eat them off the bone.

Serves: 4

Ingredients

- 1 tablespoon olive oil
- 2 teaspoons grated orange zest
- 1 tablespoon fresh orange juice
- 1 teaspoon salt
- 8 (4-ounce) lamb rib chops, trimmed

Directions

1. Combine the olive oil, orange zest, orange juice, and salt in a large ziplock bag.
2. Add the lamb to the bag and massage to coat well. Let the lamb marinate in the refrigerator for at least one hour, up to overnight.
3. Let the lamb sit at room temperature for 10 minutes prior to cooking.
4. Heat a large grill pan over medium-high heat.
5. Add the lamb to the pan and cook for 2 to 3 minutes on each side, or until done according to preference; the lamb should measure at least 145°F on a meat thermometer.
6. Serve immediately.

Serve with: *Couscous with Almonds* (page 176)

Spanish-Style Shrimp

Shrimp are often intimidating for people to cook, but I don't know why. They really are so simple to prepare and take no time at all. The best part is that the natural flavor is really mild, so they are a perfect base for really flavorful components.

Serves: 4

Ingredients

- 1 tablespoon coconut oil
- 6 garlic cloves
- 1 pound large shrimp, peeled and deveined
- ¼ teaspoon salt
- 2 tablespoons chopped fresh parsley
- Lemon wedges
- Optional: Red pepper flakes

Directions

1. Heat the coconut oil in a large skillet over medium heat. Add the garlic and cook until fragrant but not beginning to brown, about 30 seconds.
2. Add the shrimp and sauté for 4 to 5 minutes, until they've turned pink and opaque.
3. Sprinkle with the salt and parsley (and red pepper flakes if desired), add a squeeze of lemon, and serve.

Serve with: *Cauliflower Turmeric Rice* (page 164)

Mom's Wild Salmon

Salmon is my favorite fish, and this is a recipe my mom always makes in warm weather. When there are leftovers, the salmon is equally good mashed up into a salmon salad. I love this dish cooked on the rare side, especially when I use good-quality wild salmon.

Serves: 4

Ingredients

- 4 (6-ounce) wild salmon fillets
- ¼ cup maple syrup
- ¼ cup toasted sesame oil
- ¼ cup tamari (gluten-free soy sauce)
- 4 quarter-size slices fresh ginger

Directions

1. In a large ziplock bag, combine the salmon, maple syrup, sesame oil, and tamari. Lay the bag flat in the refrigerator and let the fish marinate for at least 1 hour or up to 4 hours, flipping the bag halfway through.
2. Preheat the oven to 450°F. Line a baking sheet with parchment paper or aluminum foil. Remove the salmon from the bag and place on the baking sheet, skin side down. Use a knife to make a 1-inch-long cut in each fillet; do not cut all the way through—just enough that there's room to stick a piece of the fresh ginger into each cut.
3. Bake for 12 to 15 minutes, or until the fish reaches the desired level of doneness or the center is warmed through.

Serve with: *Lemony Swiss Chard* (page 166)

Sesame Ahi Tuna Steak

Marinating anything—but especially fish—is a great, simple way to add so many flavors into a dish. I love to throw some tuna steaks into a ziplock bag in the morning and then cook them up when I get home.

Serves: 4

Ingredients

- 4 (6- to 8-ounce) ahi tuna steaks
- 2 tablespoons olive oil
- 2 tablespoons tamari (gluten-free soy sauce)
- 1 teaspoon salt
- 1 teaspoon black pepper
- 4 scallions, green parts sliced into 1-inch pieces

Directions

1. In a large ziplock bag, marinate the tuna steaks with the olive oil, tamari, salt, pepper, and scallions in the refrigerator for at least an hour, up to 3 hours.
2. Heat a medium skillet over medium-high heat.
3. Sear the tuna for 2½ minutes per side for medium-rare, 2 minutes for rare, or 3 minutes for medium.
4. Serve immediately.

Serve with: *Garlic Sweet Potato Mash* (page 185)

Baked Cod in Tomatoes

A can of tomatoes can turn any protein into something so much more! Infused with the salty taste of the capers, this dish reminds me of the ocean.

Serves: 4

Ingredients

- 1 tablespoon coconut oil
- 1 medium onion, finely chopped
- 1 (28-oz) can diced tomatoes
- 2 tablespoons capers
- 1 teaspoon salt
- 4 (6- to 8-ounce) skinless cod fillets
- 4 fresh basil leaves

Directions

1. Preheat the oven to 375°F.
2. Heat the coconut oil in a large ovenproof pan over medium-high heat.
3. Add the onion and cook until translucent, about 5 minutes.
4. Stir in the tomatoes, capers, and salt, and cook until slightly reduced, about 5 minutes.
5. Add the fish to the pan, and spoon the sauce over the top of the fish. Bake for 12 to 15 minutes, until the fish is opaque all the way through.
6. Garnish with the basil and serve immediately.

Serve with: *Zucchini Noodles Primavera* (page 173)

Steamed Cod with Ginger and Scallions

Cod lends itself well to Asian-inspired flavors. The Cold Soba Noodles make this dish extra slurpy but so good. For an easy fiber option, I like to plate this with simple sautéed spinach. The finished product looks really elegant and fools people into thinking I'm a better cook than I am!

Serves: 4

Ingredients

- 3 tablespoons rice vinegar
- 2 tablespoons tamari (gluten-free soy sauce)
- 2 tablespoons finely grated fresh ginger
- 4 (6- to 8-ounce) skinless cod fillets
- 1 teaspoon salt

Directions

1. In a large skillet over medium heat, combine the rice vinegar, tamari, and ginger. Cook for 1 minute, or until fragrant.
2. Sprinkle the cod with the salt and place in the skillet.
3. Bring the skillet to a boil, then reduce the heat to a simmer. Cover.
4. Cook the fish for 6 to 8 minutes, until it is opaque in the center.
5. Serve immediately.

Serve with: *Cold Soba Noodles* (page 180) and *Roasted Cauliflower* (page 163)

Broccoli and Cheddar Egg Muffins

This recipe is so easy, and the best part is that these muffins freeze really well, making them a great instant source of protein in the morning or at any time of day. The broccoli and Cheddar are a great base to start with, but grab whatever other vegetables or cheeses you have in the fridge.

Serves: 4

Ingredients

- 1 teaspoon coconut oil
- 1 cup raw broccoli, cut into 2-inch florets
- 8 large eggs
- ½ teaspoon salt
- ½ cup shredded Cheddar cheese

Directions

1. Preheat the oven to 375°F. Coat a 12-cup muffin tin with the coconut oil.
2. In a steamer set over boiling water, steam the broccoli, covered, for about 4 minutes.
3. Remove the broccoli from the heat, drain, and set aside to cool. In a large bowl, whisk together the eggs until fully blended and add the salt, broccoli, and Cheddar cheese.
4. Fill each muffin cup about three-quarters of the way up with the egg mixture.
5. Bake for about 10 minutes, or until the egg mixture is firm in the center.
6. Remove the egg muffins from the pan and place on a platter to cool.
7. Serve warm or enjoy cold.

Note: These freeze very well. Simply reheat them in the microwave on top of a paper towel.

Matcha-Chia Pudding

Matcha is one of my favorite flavors, so I always try to incorporate it into new recipes, even if it's just sprinkled over plain yogurt. This matcha-chia pudding combination is perfect for breakfast. I throw on some berries, and I'm good to go!

Serves: 4

Ingredients

- 2 cups almond milk
- 1 teaspoon matcha powder
- 2 teaspoons maple syrup
- ½ cups chia seeds
- Optional: Mixed berries

Directions

1. In a medium bowl, whisk together the almond milk and matcha until combined.
2. Add the maple syrup.
3. Whisk in the chia seeds.
4. Pour the mixture into a glass container and refrigerate for at least 4 hours, or overnight, until set.
5. Serve cold and top with mixed berries if desired.

FIBER

Spiced Applesauce

This is an elevated applesauce—it's perfect on its own as an afternoon snack or under a few dollops of yogurt at breakfast. I prefer it extra chunky to keep some of the apples' great texture and bite.

Serves: 4

Ingredients

- 2 pounds apples, cored, peeled, and diced
- 1 teaspoon vanilla extract
- 1 teaspoon ground cinnamon
- ½ teaspoon ground ginger
- ¼ cup water

Directions

1. In a large saucepan over high heat, combine the apples, vanilla, cinnamon, ginger, and water. Cover and cook until the fluid at the bottom begins to simmer, about 3 minutes.
2. Reduce the heat to low and continue to cook, covered, stirring with a large spoon or spatula every 5 minutes. Start mashing the apples as they soften, and continue cooking until the apples are mostly mashed, 15 to 20 minutes.
3. Remove from the heat and mash any remaining softened pieces.
4. Enjoy as is for a chunkier sauce, or purée in a blender for a silkier texture.

Sautéed Bok Choy

I love introducing people to this amazing vegetable. It keeps its crunch even when cooked and lends itself to great flavors when paired with Asian-inspired ingredients.

Serves: 4

Ingredients

- 2 tablespoons coconut oil
- 4 garlic cloves, minced
- 1 quarter-size piece fresh ginger, minced
- 1 tablespoon tamari (gluten-free soy sauce)
- 1 tablespoon water
- 1½ pounds bok choy, ends trimmed and cut into 1-inch pieces
- Optional: ¼ teaspoon red pepper flakes

Directions

1. Heat the coconut oil in a large pan over medium-high heat.
2. Add the garlic and cook, being careful not to burn it, for about 30 seconds.
3. Add the ginger and stir for a few seconds.
4. Add the tamari and water.
5. Gently add the bok choy, and red pepper flakes if desired, and combine well with the other ingredients.
6. Cook for 2 to 4 minutes, until the bok choy is easily pierced with a fork.

Roasted Brussels Sprouts

These aren't the brussels sprouts you had to choke down as a kid. Between their crispiness and their caramelization, these are a treat to eat.

Serves: 4

Ingredients

- 1 pound brussels sprouts, trimmed and halved
- 2 tablespoons olive oil
- 1 tablespoon maple syrup
- Kosher salt and freshly ground black pepper, to taste

Directions

1. Preheat the oven to 400°F. Line a baking sheet with aluminum foil.
2. In a large bowl, toss the brussels sprouts with the olive oil, maple syrup, salt, and pepper and spread onto the prepared baking sheet in a single even layer.
3. Roast for 30 to 45 minutes, stirring every 5 to 10 minutes, until crispy and browned.

Note: If there are a lot of loose leaves after halving the brussels sprouts, try adding these to the pan about 10 minutes into roasting for crispy but not overly burned leaves.

Cumin-Cinnamon Roasted Carrots

Roasting carrots is so much better than just serving them raw. You can take the lazy route here and slice them crosswise, or you can cut them in long strips (it's more work, but it makes for a fun take on French fries). Another secret: I love to burn these just a little bit; the darkened edges are my favorite part.

Serves: 4

Ingredients

- 12 carrots, cut into 1½-inch slices
- 3 tablespoons extra-virgin olive oil
- 2 teaspoons ground cumin
- 2 teaspoons ground cinnamon
- 1 teaspoon salt
- 1 teaspoon black pepper

Directions

1. Preheat the oven to 425°F.
2. In a large bowl, toss the carrots with the olive oil, cumin, cinnamon, salt, and pepper.
3. Spread the carrots over a baking sheet in a single even layer.
4. Roast until the carrots are tender and browning, 20 to 25 minutes.
5. Serve hot, warm, or at room temperature.

Roasted Cauliflower

When cauliflower is cooked right, it's delicious. There's no better way to cook cauliflower than by roasting it. I like to cut the head into very small florets so the cauliflower cooks faster and browns evenly.

Serves: 4

Ingredients

- 1 head cauliflower, cut into bite-size florets
- 1 shallot, chopped
- 2 tablespoons olive oil
- 1 teaspoon salt

Directions

1. Preheat the oven to 400°F. Line a baking sheet with aluminum foil.
2. In a large bowl, toss the cauliflower and shallot with the olive oil and sprinkle with the salt.
3. Spread the florets in a single even layer on the prepared baking sheet.
4. Roast for 40 to 50 minutes, tossing every 20 minutes, until tender and golden.

Cauliflower Turmeric Rice

I totally understand craving starches as the day wears on. What's so great about cauliflower "rice" is that it satisfies your cravings just enough to move past them for the rest of the day. This dish works as a side dish to any recipe or in the morning with eggs when there are leftovers.

Serves: 2

Ingredients

- 1 head cauliflower, washed, dried, cut into 4 even sections, and stemmed
- 1 tablespoon coconut oil
- 1 garlic clove, minced
- 2 teaspoons turmeric powder
- 1 teaspoon salt

Directions

1. In the bowl of a food processor, pulse the cauliflower until it is ricelike in texture. Work in batches if necessary; you don't want to fill the bowl more than three-quarters full.
2. Heat the coconut oil in a large skillet over medium heat.
3. Add the garlic and cook until fragrant, about 30 seconds.
4. Add the cauliflower and stir in the turmeric and salt.
5. Cover and sauté until the cauliflower pieces are easily pierced with a fork, about 5 minutes.
6. Serve hot or at room temperature.

Roasted Peppers and Onions

These peppers and onions are easy and versatile, which is why they're a great fiber option for most of the protein recipes in this book. They're especially good with Mexican cuisine; I've been known to snack on these with some guacamole while I wait for everything else to be ready.

Serves: 4

Ingredients

- 1 red bell pepper, seeded and sliced
- 1 green bell pepper, seeded and sliced
- 1 yellow bell pepper, seeded and sliced
- 1 medium red onion, sliced
- 1 tablespoon olive oil
- 2 teaspoons salt
- 1 teaspoon black pepper

Directions

1. Preheat the oven to 425°F.
2. In a large bowl, combine the peppers and onion and toss with the olive oil.
3. Sprinkle with the salt and pepper.
4. Spread the vegetables onto a baking sheet in a single even layer.
5. Roast for 10 to 15 minutes, until the vegetables are thoroughly cooked but not burned.

Lemony Swiss Chard

These greens may seem a little unruly, but when you cook them down and pair them with a bright acid like lemon, they are delicious. They're also more filling than other greens like spinach because they don't shrink down as much.

Serves: 4

Ingredients

- 2 tablespoons coconut oil
- 4 garlic cloves, minced
- 1 pound Swiss chard (about 2 large bunches), stems removed and leaves shredded
- 1 lemon
- Salt and freshly ground black pepper, to taste

Directions

1. Heat the coconut oil in a large skillet over medium heat.
2. Add the garlic and cook until golden, about 1 to 2 minutes.
3. Add the Swiss chard and cook until just tender, about 3 to 5 minutes.
4. Squeeze the lemon over the pan and cook for 1 additional minute.
5. Remove from the heat and add the salt and pepper. Serve hot.

Seared Tomatoes

This dish may not seem like anything special, but it's a great, easy addition to any meal. The juice from the tomatoes almost becomes a light broth for anything else you're cooking and adds flavor without even trying. I love combining these tomatoes with spinach and then topping them with a runny egg for an easy dinner.

Serves: 2

Ingredients

- 1 tablespoon coconut oil
- 1 garlic clove, minced
- 3 medium tomatoes, halved lengthwise
- Salt and freshly ground black pepper, to taste
- 2 tablespoons minced fresh parsley

Directions

1. Heat the coconut oil in a medium nonstick sauté pan over medium heat.
2. Cook the garlic until fragrant, about 30 seconds.
3. Arrange the tomatoes, cut side down, in the pan and cook, uncovered, until they are tender and the undersides are darkened, 10 to 15 minutes.
4. Using a wide spatula, carefully turn each tomato over. Reduce the heat to medium-low.
5. Sprinkle each tomato with the salt and pepper. Top with spoonfuls of the minced parsley.
6. Cook until brown, about 5 more minutes.

Brooke's Favorite Salad

I like nothing more than a clean, crisp salad with a bright acid flavor. I make this when we're having company over and I need a quick and easy side dish to accompany our protein. It never disappoints.

Serves: 4

Ingredients

- 1 head romaine lettuce
- 1 bunch fresh dill, finely chopped
- ½ cup pitted kalamata olives
- Juice of 1 lemon
- ½ cup olive oil
- ½ cup crumbled feta cheese

Directions

1. Cut the base of the stem off of the lettuce head. Peel off the outer leaves, leaving the heart (discard the outer leaves). Wash the lettuce thoroughly and dry with paper towels.
2. Slice the lettuce into thin strips and place in a large serving bowl.
3. Add the dill and olives and mix well. Toss with the lemon juice and olive oil.
4. Sprinkle with the feta cheese and toss well.

Creamy Kale Salad

This is one of my favorite salads. It's inspired by an amazing juice store, Juice Generation in New York City. This serves four as a side dish, or two as a main course when paired with a protein addition like the Poached and Shredded Chicken (page 146). This salad is so good that I've converted kale haters with it!

Serves: 2

Ingredients

- 1 medium avocado, pitted and peeled
- 2 tablespoons olive oil
- 2 tablespoons fresh lemon juice
- ½ teaspoon sea salt
- 4 cups curly or Russian kale, stemmed and torn into bite-size pieces
- 4 tablespoons sunflower seeds
- 2 tablespoons raisins (any color)

Directions

1. In a large bowl, mash the avocado with the olive oil, lemon juice, and salt.
2. Add the kale. Using your hands, gently massage the avocado into the kale until the kale is well coated. Let the mixture sit for 20 minutes.
3. Sprinkle the sunflower seeds and raisins over the kale and avocado mixture.
4. Serve immediately.

Note: Don't skip out on massaging the kale! It seems weird, but it helps make the kale easier to eat and digest.

Summer Salad

I eat a lot of salads; it's kind of a professional responsibility. This salad was inspired by one my husband and I used to order all the time. It was simple, but it was so good that we would fight over it. So I decided to make my own so there would always be enough for both of us.

Serves: 4

Ingredients

- 4 medium tomatoes, diced
- 1 large cucumber, seeded and diced
- 2 red bell peppers, seeded and diced
- ½ cup olive oil
- ¼ cup red wine vinegar
- ½ cup crumbled feta cheese
- Salt and freshly ground black pepper, to taste

Directions

1. In a large bowl, combine the tomatoes, cucumber, and peppers.
2. In a small bowl, whisk together the olive oil and red wine vinegar until combined.
3. Pour the dressing over the vegetables and toss well.
4. Add salt and pepper and top with the feta cheese.

Spaghetti Squash Pizza Bowl

I brought this dish to a friend's house for a holiday dinner once and all the men at the table couldn't stop raving about it. That's when I knew I was really onto something. Getting these guys to ask for seconds of spaghetti squash was hilarious, but it's true—this really tastes like an indulgence.

Serves: 4

Ingredients

- 1 medium spaghetti squash, halved lengthwise and seeds scooped out
- 1 (24-ounce) jar tomato sauce (no sugar added)
- 1 cup ricotta cheese
- ¾ cup shredded mozzarella cheese
- ¼ cup grated Parmesan cheese

Directions

1. Preheat the oven to 400°F. Line a baking sheet and a glass baking pan with aluminum foil.
2. Place the spaghetti squash on the prepared baking sheet flesh side down.
3. Bake for 30 to 45 minutes, until you can easily poke a fork into the squash.
4. Flip the squash over and let cool for 10 minutes. Then, using a fork, "rake" the squash to create the noodles, scooping them into a large bowl.
5. Add the tomato sauce and ricotta and mozzarella cheeses and mix until well combined.
6. Add the squash and sauce mixture to the prepared glass baking pan and bake for about 15 minutes.
7. Sprinkle with the Parmesan cheese and bake for another 5 to 10 minutes, until the cheese is slightly golden brown.
8. Serve warm.

Note: If the spaghetti squash is too tough to halve at first, microwave it for 2 to 3 minutes to help soften it.

Veggie "Pizza"

This will satisfy any pizza craving and still counts as your fiber—not bad, right? The mushrooms are sturdy and have a firm texture, so they make a great replacement for your dough. Simply add some ground beef or plain diced chicken to the spinach for an all-in-one dish.

Serves: 4

Ingredients

- 1 teaspoon olive oil
- 1 tablespoon coconut oil
- 2 cups baby spinach
- 4 portobello mushrooms, stems removed
- ½ cup tomato sauce (no sugar added)
- 1 cup shredded mozzarella cheese

Directions

1. Preheat the oven to 400°F. Line a baking sheet with aluminum foil and grease with the olive oil.
2. Heat the coconut oil in a medium pan over medium heat. Add the spinach.
3. Cook the spinach until completely wilted and cooked through, about 3 to 5 minutes.
4. Transfer the spinach to a paper towel–lined plate to absorb the extra water. Set aside.
5. Place the mushrooms on the prepared baking sheet, and spoon about 2 tablespoons of the tomato sauce into each cap.
6. Bake for 20 minutes.
7. Portion the spinach and mozzarella cheese into each cap, and bake for another 5 minutes, or until the cheese is melted.
8. Serve immediately.

Zucchini Noodles Primavera

Zucchini noodles, aka zoodles, make eating your veggies fun again. These noodles are sturdy enough for toppings like the primavera-style sauce I've paired them with here. Any simple protein will go great with this, and the combination will be an easy, homey meal that's loaded with fiber.

Serves: 4

Ingredients

- 2 tablespoons coconut oil, divided
- 4 medium zucchini, spiralized with a ⅛-inch spacing blade or cut into long strips with a vegetable peeler
- 1 garlic clove
- 1 cup grape or cherry tomatoes, quartered
- 1 teaspoon salt
- Juice of 1 lemon
- 3 to 4 tablespoons Parmesan cheese

Directions

1. Heat 1 tablespoon of the coconut oil in a large skillet over medium heat. Add the zoodles (the zucchini strips) and cook until tender but still crunchy, 2 to 3 minutes.
2. Remove the pan from the heat and let it sit for 1 to 3 minutes so the zucchini can release their extra moisture.
3. Drain the zoodles through a colander and place on a paper towel–lined plate to absorb any extra liquid.
4. Wipe the skillet clean and heat the remaining 1 tablespoon coconut oil over medium heat. Add the garlic and sauté until fragrant, 30 seconds.
5. Add the tomatoes and salt and reduce the heat to a simmer. Cook until the juices from the tomatoes come out, 4 to 5 minutes. Remove from the heat.
6. Return the zoodles to the pan and add the lemon juice and Parmesan cheese. Gently combine.
7. Serve immediately.

STARCH

Black Rice with Coconut Milk

I love traditional black rice pudding recipes. Sadly for me, they're often loaded with sugar. So I set off to see if I could make my own version, but as a side dish instead of a dessert option. The result turned out to be extra chewy and very satisfying.

Serves: 4

Ingredients

- 1 cup black rice
- ¼ teaspoon salt
- 1 (13½-ounce) can unsweetened full-fat coconut milk

Directions

1. In a large saucepan over high heat, combine the black rice, salt, and coconut milk and bring to a boil.
2. Reduce the heat to a simmer and cover. Cook until the rice is tender but still chewy, about 40 minutes.
3. Remove the rice from the heat and let it sit for 10 minutes, stirring occasionally.
4. Serve warm or at room temperature.

Tahini Brown Rice

In this dish we combine two starches into one, merging the sweetness of the sweet potato with the nutty flavor of the brown rice. Adding the tahini is the way to meld all the flavors together. To make the dish extra pretty to serve, top it with some fresh herbs like parsley if you have any extra around. Just watch your portions here—this is way easy to overeat!

Serves: 4

Ingredients

- 1 medium sweet potato, peeled and cut into 1-inch cubes
- 2 teaspoons olive oil
- 1 teaspoon salt
- 1 cup brown rice, cooked according to package instructions
- 2 tablespoons tahini

Directions

1. Preheat the oven to 400°F.
2. Place the sweet potato on a roasting pan or baking sheet and coat well with the olive oil and salt.
3. Roast for 25 to 30 minutes, until tender.
4. Carefully transfer the sweet potato to a medium bowl and combine with the brown rice. Pour the tahini over the top and mix well.
5. Serve hot or at room temperature.

Couscous with Almonds

I have always enjoyed the texture of couscous, plus it's an easy grain to flavor simply for a great starch option. It's even delicious plain, with just some of a fat option like butter or oil and a bit of salt. The almonds give this dish a crunch that makes it even more satisfying.

Serves: 4

Ingredients

- ¾ cup water
- ½ cup couscous
- 2 tablespoons unsalted butter
- ½ medium onion, finely chopped
- 2 tablespoons finely chopped fresh parsley
- ¼ cup slivered almonds
- Salt, to taste

Directions

1. In a small saucepan, bring the water to a boil.
2. Add the couscous and stir once, then cover and remove from the heat. Let the couscous sit for 5 minutes to cook.
3. Heat the butter in a separate small saucepan over medium heat. Add the onion and cook until translucent, about 5 minutes. Remove from the heat.
4. Add the parsley to the cooked onion and mix well.
5. Fluff the couscous with a fork and mix in the parsley and onion mixture and salt. Sprinkle the almonds over the top of the couscous.
6. Serve warm or at room temperature.

Coconutty Quinoa

For a while, I really didn't like quinoa, no matter how many times I made it. As a healthy eater, this judgment felt wrong—like hating kale! So I switched my approach, first by rinsing it well and then by cooking it in chicken broth. I liked it much better and started experimenting even more. Now, I swear by cooking it in coconut milk and topping it with some lime zest.

Serves: 6

Ingredients

- 1 cup quinoa
- 1 tablespoon coconut oil
- 1 cup unsweetened full-fat coconut milk
- 1 cup water
- 1 teaspoon kosher salt
- 2 limes, halved
- 1 teaspoon lime zest

Directions

1. Place the quinoa in a fine-mesh strainer and rinse with cold water until the water runs clear. Set aside.
2. Heat the coconut oil in a medium saucepan over medium heat. Add the quinoa and cook, stirring often, until golden in color, about 5 minutes.
3. Add the coconut milk, water, and salt and stir to combine.
4. Bring to a boil, then reduce the heat to a simmer and cover.
5. Cook until the liquid has evaporated and the quinoa appears to have a halo around each seed, 20 to 25 minutes.
6. Let the quinoa sit, covered, for 10 minutes.
7. Squeeze the limes over the quinoa, add the zest, and fluff with a fork.

Fresh Quinoa Salad

Once I figured out how to make quinoa taste good, I realized it was a great starch choice for a grainlike salad. The mint and lime make this dish so refreshing, and I love it even more the next day as leftovers because the flavors get even stronger.

Serves: 4

Ingredients

- 1 cup quinoa
- 1¾ cups vegetable or chicken broth
- 1 tablespoon fresh lime juice
- 2 tablespoons extra-virgin olive oil
- Kosher salt and freshly ground black pepper, to taste
- 8 large fresh mint leaves, finely chopped
- Optional: ¼ cup pomegranate seeds

Directions

1. Place the quinoa in a fine-mesh strainer and rinse with cold water until the water runs clear.
2. Add the quinoa and broth to a medium saucepan over high heat and bring to a boil.
3. Reduce the heat to a simmer, cover, and cook until the liquid is absorbed, 10 to 15 minutes. Remove from the heat and let the quinoa sit, covered, for an additional 5 minutes.
4. In a large bowl, gently whisk together the lime juice and olive oil.
5. Fluff the quinoa with a fork and add to the large bowl. Add the salt and pepper, mix gently, and top with the mint.
6. Serve the quinoa at room temperature or cold. Top with pomegranate seeds if desired.

Farro with Pistachios

I like to experiment with different high-fiber grains in the kitchen, and farro is my latest obsession. Since it's got a natural nutty flavor to it, pairing it with chopped pistachios seems like the right move.

Serves: 4

Ingredients

- 2 cups water
- 1 cup semi-pearled farro
- ½ teaspoon salt
- 1½ teaspoons coconut oil
- 1 medium onion, finely chopped
- 1 cup shelled and salted pistachios, chopped
- 1 tablespoon red wine vinegar

Directions

1. In a large saucepan, bring the water, farro, and salt to a boil. Reduce the heat to a simmer, and cook, stirring occasionally, until tender, 15 to 20 minutes.
2. Transfer the farro to a large bowl, draining the extra fluid if necessary.
3. Heat the coconut oil in a small skillet over medium-high heat. Add the onion and cook until translucent, about 5 minutes. Remove from the heat.
4. Add the onion to the farro and mix in the pistachios.
5. Top with the red wine vinegar and toss until well combined.

Cold Soba Noodles

It's not always easy to find healthy pasta dishes, but this dish passes the test. Soba noodles have more protein and fiber than regular noodles do, so these noodles count as a starch instead of an intentional indulgence.

Serves: 4

Ingredients

- 8 ounces soba or buckwheat noodles
- 1 cup chicken broth
- ¼ cup tamari (gluten-free soy sauce)
- 1 teaspoon grated fresh ginger
- 1 teaspoon honey
- 1 tablespoon water

Directions

1. Rinse the noodles well in a colander.
2. Fill a large pot with water and bring to a boil.
3. Add the noodles and bring the water back to a boil. Cook until the noodles are soft but not mushy, 5 to 8 minutes, and then drain immediately. Rinse the noodles in cold water and transfer to a serving bowl.
4. In a small bowl, whisk together the broth, tamari, ginger, honey, and water.
5. Pour the sauce over the noodles and gently toss.

Socca Bread

This bread is similar to a pita. Since it's made from chickpea flour, it also has protein and fiber, but it still counts as a starch here. It's great as a side for a salad or as a base for a healthy homemade pizza.

Serves: 4

Ingredients

- 1 cup chickpea flour
- 1 teaspoon salt
- 1 cup water
- 2 tablespoons olive oil
- 1 tablespoon coconut oil

Directions

1. In a medium bowl, combine the chickpea flour and salt.
2. Add the water and whisk until there are no lumps left.
3. Slowly pour in the olive oil and mix. Cover with a dishcloth or plastic wrap and set aside while the oven heats.
4. Place a cast-iron skillet in the oven and heat the oven to 450°F.
5. Once the oven reaches 450°F, carefully remove the skillet from the oven and grease with the coconut oil, swirling the pan to coat it.
6. Pour the batter into the skillet and bake for 12 to 15 minutes, until the center of the "bread" is firm and cooked through.

Cheesy Herbed Popcorn

You can never go wrong with popcorn, but it *is* easy to overeat it. That's why I add strong flavors like Parmesan cheese and garlic butter to make for a more satisfying snack—the intense flavors make it easier to watch your portions.

Serves: 4

Ingredients

- 3 tablespoons coconut oil
- ⅓ cup popcorn kernels (GMO-free)
- 2 tablespoons salted butter
- 1 garlic clove, minced
- 1 tablespoon dried oregano
- ¼ cup grated Parmesan cheese

Directions

1. Add the coconut oil and a few popcorn kernels to a large saucepan over medium-high heat and cover until you hear the kernels pop.
2. Add the rest of the kernels and cover the pan again.
3. Cook the kernels, shaking the pan regularly, until the popping slows down, 2 to 3 minutes. Uncover and remove from the heat.
4. Melt the butter in a small saucepan over medium heat.
5. Add the garlic and oregano and cook until fragrant, about 30 seconds.
6. Remove from the heat and pour the garlic butter over the popcorn.
7. Sprinkle the Parmesan cheese over the top and toss until the popcorn is well coated.
8. Serve immediately.

Corn Salad

Nothing screams summer to me more than fresh corn. My family loves to eat it right off the cob, but I always end up messing around with the leftovers to make a yummy salad-type dish. This dish is almost like a corn salsa. I love using it as a topper for Poached and Shredded Chicken (page 146) or anything that needs a boost of flavor, like a simple salad.

Serves: 4

Ingredients

- 4 ears corn, shucked, boiled, and cooled
- 1 red bell pepper, seeded and diced
- 2 celery stalks, diced
- 1 cup cherry or grape tomatoes, halved
- 2 tablespoons olive oil
- ¼ teaspoon salt
- Juice of 1 lime

Directions

1. In a large bowl, combine the cooled corn kernels with the pepper, celery, and tomatoes.
2. Toss with the olive oil, salt, and lime juice.
3. Serve cold or at room temperature.

Pesto Roasted Potatoes

I'll put pesto on almost anything. I love it on eggs, sliced turkey, or any vegetable. Here it adds brightness and flavor to simple roasted potatoes.

Serves: 8

Ingredients

- 2 pounds small red or white potatoes, cut into 1-inch cubes
- 2 tablespoons basil pesto (homemade or store-bought)
- 2 teaspoons kosher salt
- 2 tablespoons Parmesan cheese

Directions

1. Preheat the oven to 400°F.
2. In a large bowl, toss together the potatoes and pesto until the potatoes are well coated.
3. Spread the potatoes onto a large baking sheet in a single even layer and sprinkle with the salt.
4. Bake for 45 minutes, flipping once or twice with a spatula to ensure even cooking.
5. Sprinkle the Parmesan cheese over the potatoes and return them to the oven for an additional 10 minutes, or until they can be easily pierced by a fork.
6. Serve immediately.

Garlic Sweet Potato Mash

I wouldn't normally think to match garlic with sweet flavors, but this dish just works. It's sweet and creamy with that great punch of garlic flavor, and it makes for a fantastic starch side to any protein or fiber dish.

Serves: 4

Ingredients

- 4 medium sweet potatoes, peeled
- 4 garlic cloves, minced
- 1 teaspoon kosher salt
- ¼ cup whole milk, plus more as needed

Directions

1. Bring a large pot of water to a boil.
2. Place the sweet potatoes in the water and bring back to a boil. Cook until tender, 20 to 30 minutes.
3. On a cutting board, sprinkle the minced garlic with the salt and form into a tidy pile. Flatten the pile with the blunt side of a knife and press and scrape the knife at an angle to flatten the garlic. Work the garlic back into a tidy pile and repeat, pressing and scraping the knife through the pile for 2 to 3 minutes until you have a smooth paste. Set aside.
4. Drain the sweet potatoes and return them back to the pot.
5. Add the garlic paste and milk.
6. Using an immersion blender, blend to reach your desired texture. Add more milk if necessary.
7. Serve warm.

Sweet Potato Wedges

I don't trust people who don't like French fries. Here's a great version to make at home—these fries don't count as an intentional indulgence since they're made from sweet potatoes and baked in the oven.

Serves: 3 to 4

Ingredients

- 3 large sweet potatoes, peeled and cut into 1-inch-wide wedges
- 2 tablespoons olive oil
- 2 teaspoons paprika
- ½ teaspoon cayenne pepper
- ½ teaspoon garlic powder
- 1 teaspoon salt
- ½ teaspoon black pepper

Directions

1. Preheat the oven to 400°F. Line a large baking sheet with aluminum foil or parchment paper.
2. In a large bowl, toss the sweet potatoes with the olive oil until well coated.
3. In a small bowl, combine the paprika, cayenne, garlic powder, salt, and pepper.
4. Pour the spice mix over the sweet potatoes and mix well.
5. Place the potato wedges on the prepared baking sheet.
6. Roast, flipping every so often, for about 30 minutes, until soft.

Butternut Squash

The natural sweetness of this winter squash comes out even more when it's roasted well. Those burned little ends are always my favorite bites. I like to keep the flavors simple to let the naturally delicious flavor of the squash shine.

Serves: 4

Ingredients

- 1 medium butternut squash (about 2 pounds), peeled, seeded, and cut into 1-inch cubes
- 2 tablespoons olive oil
- 1 teaspoon kosher salt
- 1 teaspoon black pepper

Directions

1. Preheat the oven to 400°F. Line a baking sheet with aluminum foil.
2. In a large bowl, toss the butternut squash with the olive oil, salt, and pepper.
3. Spread the squash onto the prepared baking sheet in a single even layer.
4. Roast for 25 to 30 minutes, stirring occasionally, until tender and golden.

Salt and Vinegar Chickpeas

For some reason, regular salted potato chips don't tempt me. I can easily decline them without feeling any deprivation. It's a whole other story with salt and vinegar chips, though. Something about the combination makes them irresistible to me. To capture that same salt and vinegar taste in a healthier package, I use chickpeas. While chickpeas are considered a starch in this plan, they also contain fiber and protein, making them a much more wholesome option than traditional salt and vinegar chips.

Serves: 6

Ingredients

- 2 (16-ounce) cans chickpeas, rinsed well and drained
- 3 cups white distilled vinegar
- 2 tablespoons olive oil
- 2 tablespoons salt

Directions

1. Preheat the oven to 400°F.
2. In a medium pot, combine the chickpeas and vinegar and bring to a boil. Remove the chickpeas from the heat and let them sit for 30 minutes.
3. Drain the chickpeas. Transfer the chickpeas to a large bowl and toss with the olive oil and salt.
4. Spread the chickpeas on a baking sheet and bake, stirring occasionally, for 30 to 40 minutes, until browned and crunchy.

Building a Meal

To make it even easier for you to think of great meal combinations, here are some of the proteins, fibers, and starches that I love to mix and match. These are just suggestions—remember that a protein and a fiber is all you need to have a complete plate. Don't overthink it!

Protein: Asian-Inspired Grilled Chicken (page 144)
Fiber: Sautéed Bok Choy (page 160)
Starch: Fresh Quinoa Salad (page 178)

Protein: Chili-Lime Chicken Strips (page 145)
Fiber: Roasted Brussels Sprouts (page 161)
Starch: Fresh Quinoa Salad (page 178)

Protein: Poached and Shredded Chicken (page 146)
Fiber: Creamy Kale Salad (page 169)

Protein: Turmeric-Almond Chicken Fingers (page 147)
Fiber: Cumin-Cinnamon Roasted Carrots (page 162)

Protein: Pesto Turkey Burger (page 148)
Fiber: Brooke's Favorite Salad (page 168)
Starch: Tahini Brown Rice (page 175)

Protein: Turkey Lettuce Tacos (page 149)
Fiber: Roasted Peppers and Onions (page 165)

Protein: Spiced Beef Burger (page 150)
Starch: Sweet Potato Wedges (page 186)

Protein: Orange-Glazed Lamb Chops (page 151)
Starch: Couscous with Almonds (page 176)

Protein: Spanish-Style Shrimp (page 152)
Fiber: Cauliflower Turmeric Rice (page 164)
Starch: Pesto Roasted Potatoes (page 184)

Protein: Mom's Wild Salmon (page 153)
Fiber: Lemony Swiss Chard (page 166)

Protein: Sesame Ahi Tuna Steak (page 154)
Starch: Garlic Sweet Potato Mash (page 185)

Protein: Baked Cod in Tomatoes (page 155)
Fiber: Zucchini Noodles Primavera (page 173)

Protein: Steamed Cod with Ginger and Scallions (page 156)
Fiber: Roasted Cauliflower (page 163)
Starch: Cold Soba Noodles (page 180)

Shopping List and Serving Size Guide

After the options, I added the ideal kinds for you to look for. Whenever you can meet that ideal criteria, that's great, but these options aren't always easy to find. Just do your best.

- ☐ Dairy (look for grass-fed, organic, full-fat, and unsweetened)
    - ☐ Cottage cheese   ½ cup
    - ☐ Cheese   1 ounce
        - ☐ Cheddar
        - ☐ Feta
        - ☐ Mozzarella
        - ☐ Parmesan
        - ☐ Ricotta   ¼ cup
    - ☐ Milk   1 cup
        - ☐ Milk alternatives
            - ☐ Almond milk
            - ☐ Coconut milk
        - ☐ Yogurt*   5–7 ounces
- ☐ Eggs (look for pastured and organic)   2–3 whole eggs
- ☐ Nuts and seeds
    - ☐ Almonds   ⅓ cup or 1½ ounces
    - ☐ Almond meal   ⅓ cup or 1½ ounces
    - ☐ Cashews   ⅓ cup or 1½ ounces
    - ☐ Chia seeds/pudding   2 tablespoons seeds, ½ cup pudding

*For items marked with an asterisk, see recommended brands on page 196.

☐ Pecans   ⅓ cup or 1½ ounces
☐ Pistachios   ⅓ cup or 1½ ounces
☐ Sunflower seeds   ⅓ cup or 1½ ounces
☐ Walnuts   ⅓ cup or 1½ ounces
☐ Nut butters (look for unsweetened
   varieties)*   2 tablespoons
   ☐ Almond butter
   ☐ Cashew butter
   ☐ Peanut butter
☐ Plant-based protein options (look for organic and non-GMO)
   ☐ Beans   ½ cup
   ☐ Hemp seeds   2 tablespoons
   ☐ Hummus   2 tablespoons
   ☐ Spirulina   ½ cup
   ☐ Tofu   6 ounces
☐ Poultry (look for free-range, pastured,
   and organic)   6 ounces
   ☐ Chicken (white or dark meat)
   ☐ Turkey (white or dark meat)
☐ Red meat (look for grass-fed
   and organic)   6 ounces
   ☐ Beef
   ☐ Bison
   ☐ Lamb
   ☐ Pork
☐ Seafood (look for wild-caught and
   sustainably fished)   6 ounces
   ☐ Cod
   ☐ Salmon
   ☐ Shellfish
   ☐ Shrimp
   ☐ Sole
   ☐ Tuna

FIBER

Whenever possible, try to find organic versions.

- ☐ Fruit (This list includes low-sugar fruits; all fruit is good, but these are the best ones.)
  - ☐ Apples   1 medium
  - ☐ Berries   ½ cup
  - ☐ Grapefruit   ½ whole fruit
  - ☐ Grapes   ½ cup
  - ☐ Honeydew, cantaloupe   ½ cup
  - ☐ Lemons, limes   unlimited
  - ☐ Oranges, tangerines   1 whole fruit
  - ☐ Clementines   2 whole fruits
  - ☐ Peaches, nectarines, plums   1 whole fruit
  - ☐ Pears   1 medium
  - ☐ Pomegranate seeds   ¼ cup
  - ☐ Tomato   1 whole fruit
- ☐ Vegetables
  - ☐ Artichoke   1 large
  - ☐ Asparagus   unlimited
  - ☐ Bok choy   unlimited
  - ☐ Broccoli   unlimited
  - ☐ Brussels sprouts   unlimited
  - ☐ Cabbage   unlimited
  - ☐ Carrots   unlimited
  - ☐ Cauliflower   unlimited
  - ☐ Celery   unlimited
  - ☐ Cucumber   unlimited
  - ☐ Eggplant   1 cup
  - ☐ Green beans   1 cup
  - ☐ Leafy greens, spinach, kale,
    Swiss chard, collard greens   unlimited
  - ☐ Lettuce (all kinds)   unlimited
  - ☐ Mushrooms   1 cup
  - ☐ Onions   1 cup raw, ½ cup cooked
  - ☐ Peppers   1 cup
  - ☐ Spaghetti squash   1 cup
  - ☐ Zucchini, summer squash   1 cup

STARCH (NO SUGAR ADDED)

Always try to get whole-grain options whenever possible.

☐ Butternut squash	½ cup
☐ Chickpeas	½ cup
☐ Corn	½ cup, 1 small ear
☐ Farro	½ cup
☐ Granola*	½ cup
☐ High-fiber crackers*	1 serving
☐ Noodles (soba or whole grain)*	2 ounces or ½ cup (cooked)
☐ Peas	½ cup
☐ Popcorn*	2 cups
☐ Quinoa	½ cup (cooked)
☐ Red or white potato	1 small or ½ cup
☐ Rice (white, brown, or black)	½ cup (cooked)
☐ Sweet potato	1 small or ½ large
☐ Tortilla/wrap	1 small
☐ Multigrain bread*	1 slice

FAT

☐ Avocado	½ avocado
☐ Butter*	1 tablespoon
☐ Coconut oil	1 tablespoon
☐ Ghee	1 tablespoon
☐ Guacamole	2 tablespoons
☐ Olive oil	1 tablespoon
☐ Sesame oil, plain or toasted	2 tablespoons

COOKING ESSENTIALS

☐ Hot sauce	☐ Rice vinegar
☐ Mustard (no sugar added)	☐ Salsa (no sugar added)
☐ Pesto	☐ Tahini
☐ Red wine vinegar	☐ Tamari (gluten-free soy sauce)

☐ Tomato paste
☐ Tomato sauce (no sugar added)
☐ Canned diced tomatoes

☐ Balsamic vinegar
☐ White distilled vinegar
☐ Vegetable or chicken broth

FRESH OR DRIED HERBS, SPICES, SEASONINGS

☐ Basil
☐ Cayenne pepper
☐ Chili powder
☐ Cinnamon
☐ Cumin
☐ Dill
☐ Garlic
☐ Garlic powder
☐ Ginger
☐ Mint
☐ Onion powder

☐ Oregano
☐ Paprika
☐ Parsley
☐ Pepper
☐ Red pepper flakes
☐ Salt
☐ Scallion
☐ Sesame seeds
☐ Shallot
☐ Turmeric
☐ Vanilla extract

MISCELLANEOUS

☐ Capers
☐ Dandelion root tea*
☐ Dark chocolate*
☐ Jerky

☐ Kalamata olives
☐ Kale chips*
☐ Matcha
☐ Raisins

SWEETENERS

☐ Honey

☐ Maple syrup

Brands I Love

The supermarket is loaded with tons of options, but everyone is always asking for my favorite products. So here's a list of them, which I think you'll love, too.

P: Protein   **F:** Fiber   **S:** Starch

CEREALS (S)

☐ Nature's Path Qi'a cereal
☐ WholeMe Clusters

☐ Purely Elizabeth Ancient Grain Granola

YOGURT (P)

☐ Fage

☐ Siggi's

NUT BUTTER (P)

☐ Barney Butter
☐ Justin's

☐ NuttZo

CHIA (P)

☐ The Chia Co chia pods

☐ The Chia Co chia seeds

SNACKS

☐ Brad's kale chips (F)
☐ Simple Mills almond flour crackers (S)

☐ Mary's Gone Crackers (S)
☐ Quinn Snacks popcorn (S)

SNACK BARS

☐ Elemental Superfood Seedbar
☐ Health Warrior Chia Bar
☐ Kind

☐ Lärabar
☐ Perfect Bar
☐ Raw Crunch
☐ Wild Zora

BREAD/WRAPS/PASTA (S)

- ☐ Ancient Harvest pasta
- ☐ Food for Life Ezekiel 4:9 organic sprouted whole-grain bread
- ☐ Cappello's almond flour pasta
- ☐ Food for Life Ezekiel 4:9 sprouted whole-grain tortillas
- ☐ La Tortilla Factory wraps

CHOCOLATE

- ☐ Eating Evolved
- ☐ Green & Black's
- ☐ Hu Kitchen
- ☐ Nib Mor
- ☐ Sweetriot

DRINKS

- ☐ Alvita dandelion root tea

BUTTERS

- ☐ Kerrygold

References

Chapter 1: Diet Takedown

The Global Healthy Weight Registry. 2017. *Food & Brand Lab, Cornell University.* http://foodpsychology.cornell.edu/discoveries/global-healthy-weight-registry

Lowe, Michael R., Sapna D. Doshi, Shawn N. Katterman, and Emily H. Feig. 2013. "Dieting and Restrained Eating as Prospective Predictors of Weight Gain." *Frontiers in Psychology* 4. doi:10.3389/fpsyg.2013.00577

Thaiss, Christoph A., Shlomik Itav, Daphna Rothschild, Mariska T. Meijer, Maayan Levy, Claudia Moresi, Lenka Dohnalová, et al. 2016. "Persistent Microbiome Alterations Modulate the Rate of Post-Dieting Weight Regain." *Nature* 540 (7634): 544–551. doi:10.1038/nature20796

Chapter 4: The Rules

Rule #1: Eat Protein and Fiber at Every Meal

Clark, Michelle J., and Joanne L. Slavin. 2013. "The Effect of Fiber on Satiety and Food Intake: A Systematic Review." *Journal of the American College of Nutrition* 32 (3): 200–211. doi:10.1080/07315724.2013.791194

Desai, Mahesh S., Anna M. Seekatz, Nicole M. Koropatkin, Nobuhiko Kamada, Christina A. Hickey, Mathis Wolter, Nicholas A. Pudlo, et al. 2016. "A Dietary Fiber-Deprived Gut Microbiota Degrades the Colonic Mucus Barrier and Enhances Pathogen Susceptibility." *Cell* 167 (5): 1339–1353.e21. doi:10.1016/j.cell.2016.10.043

Dhiman, T. R., G. R. Anand, L. D. Satter, and M. W. Pariza. 1999. "Conjugated Linoleic Acid Content of Milk from Cows Fed Different Diets." *Journal of Dairy Science* 82 (10): 2146–2156. doi:10.3168/jds.s0022-0302(99)75458-5

Leidy, Heather J., Minghua Tang, Cheryl L. H. Armstrong, Carmen B. Martin, and Wayne W. Campbell. 2010. "The Effects of Consuming Frequent, Higher Protein Meals on Appetite and Satiety During Weight Loss in Overweight/Obese Men." *Obesity* 19 (4): 818–824. doi:10.1038/oby.2010.203

Lin, Yi, Inge Huybrechts, Carine Vereecken, Theodora Mouratidou, Jara Valtueña, Mathilde Kersting, Marcela González-Gross, et al. 2014. "Dietary Fiber Intake and Its Association with Indicators of Adiposity and Serum Biomarkers in European Adolescents: The HELENA Study." *European Journal of Nutrition* 54 (5): 771–782. doi:10.1007/s00394-014-0756-2

Luft, Andreas R., Manuel M. Buitrago, Thomas Ringer, Johannes Dichgans, and Jörg B. Schulz. 2004. "Motor Skill Learning Depends on Protein Synthesis in Motor Cortex After Training." *Journal of Neuroscience* 24 (29): 6515–6520. doi:10.1523/jneurosci.1034-04.2004

Pariza, Michael W. 2004. "Perspective on the Safety and Effectiveness of Conjugated Linoleic Acid." *American Journal of Clinical Nutrition* 79 (6): 1132S–1136S.

"Seafood Recommendations from the Seafood Watch Program at the Monterey Bay Aquarium." 2017. *Seafood Watch.* https://www.seafoodwatch.org/seafood-recommendations

Weigle, David S., Patricia A. Breen, Colleen C. Matthys, Holly S. Callahan, Kaatje E. Meeuws, Verna R. Burden, and Jonathan Q. Purnell. 2005. "A High-Protein Diet Induces Sustained Reductions in Appetite, Ad Libitum Caloric Intake, and Body Weight Despite Compensatory Changes in Diurnal Plasma Leptin and Ghrelin Concentrations." *American Journal of Clinical Nutrition* 82 (1): 41–48.

Rule #2: Check Your Starches

Bazzano, Lydia A., Tian Hu, Kristi Reynolds, Lu Yao, Calynn Bunol, Yanxi Liu, Chung-Shiuan Chen, et al. 2014. "Effects of Low-Carbohydrate and Low-Fat Diets." *Annals of Internal Medicine* 161 (5): 309. doi:10.7326/m14-0180

Foster, Gary D., Holly R. Wyatt, James O. Hill, Angela P. Makris, Diane L. Rosenbaum, Carrie Brill, Richard I. Stein, et al. 2010. "Weight and Metabolic Outcomes After 2 Years on a Low-Carbohydrate Versus Low-Fat Diet." *Annals of Internal Medicine* 153 (3): 147. doi:10.7326/0003-4819-153-3-201008030-00005

"Glycemic Index and Glycemic Load for 100+ Foods." 2015. *Harvard Health Publications.* http://www.health.harvard.edu/diseases-and-conditions/glycemic_index_and_glycemic_load_for_100_foods

Lennerz, Belinda S., David C. Alsop, Laura M. Holsen, Emily Stern, Rafael Rojas, Cara B. Ebbeling, Jill M. Goldstein, et al. 2013. "Effects of Dietary Glycemic Index on Brain Regions Related to Reward and Craving in Men." *American Journal of Clinical Nutrition* 98 (3): 641–647. doi:10.3945/ajcn.113.064113

Ludwig, David S., Joseph A. Majzoub, Ahmad Al-Zahrani, Gerald E. Dallal, Isaac Blanco, and Susan B. Roberts. 1999. "High Glycemic Index Foods, Overeating, and Obesity." *Pediatrics* 103 (3): e26–e26. doi:10.1542/peds.103.3.e26

Rule #3: Clock Your Meals

Alperet, Derrick Johnston, Lesley M. Butler, Woon-Puay Koh, Jian-Min Yuan, and Rob M. van Dam. 2017. "Influence of Temperate, Subtropical, and Tropical Fruit Consumption on Risk of Type 2 Diabetes in an Asian Population." *American Journal of Clinical Nutrition* 105 (3): 736–745. doi:10.3945/ajcn.116.147090

Bo, S., M. Fadda, A. Castiglione, G. Ciccone, A. De Francesco, D. Fedele, A. Guggino, et al. 2015. "Is the Timing of Caloric Intake Associated with Variation in Diet-Induced Thermogenesis and in the Metabolic Pattern? A Randomized Cross-Over Study." *International Journal of Obesity* 39 (12): 1689–1695. doi:10.1038/ijo.2015.138

Chaix, Amandine, Amir Zarrinpar, Phuong Miu, and Satchidananda Panda. 2014. "Time-Restricted Feeding Is a Preventative and Therapeutic Intervention Against Diverse Nutritional Challenges." *Cell Metabolism* 20 (6): 991–1005. doi:10.1016/j.cmet.2014.11.001

Rule #4: Eat Fat

Assunção, Monica L., Haroldo S. Ferreira, Aldenir F. dos Santos, Cyro R. Cabral, and Telma M. M. T. Florêncio. 2009. "Effects of Dietary Coconut Oil on the Biochemical and Anthropometric Profiles of Women Presenting Abdominal Obesity." *Lipids* 44 (7): 593–601. doi:10.1007/s11745-009-3306-6

Golomb, Beatrice A., Sabrina Koperski, and Halbert L. White. 2012. "Association Between More Frequent Chocolate Consumption and Lower Body Mass Index." *Archives of Internal Medicine* 172 (6): 519. doi:10.1001/archinternmed.2011.2100

He, Ka, Anwar Merchant, Eric B. Rimm, Bernard A. Rosner, Meir J. Stampfer, Walter C. Willett, and Alberto Ascherio. 2003. "Dietary Fat Intake and Risk of Stroke in Male US Healthcare Professionals: 14 Year Prospective Cohort Study." *BMJ* 327 (7418): 777–782. doi:10.1136/bmj.327.7418.777

Norris, Leigh E., Angela L. Collene, Michelle L. Asp, Jason C. Hsu, Li-Fen Liu, Julia R. Richardson, Dongmei Li, et al. 2009. "Comparison of Dietary Conjugated Linoleic Acid with Safflower Oil on Body Composition in Obese Postmenopausal Women with Type 2 Diabetes Mellitus." *American Journal of Clinical Nutrition* 90 (3): 468–476. doi:10.3945/ajcn.2008.27371

Siri-Tarino, P. W, Q. Sun, F. B. Hu, and R. M. Krauss. 2010. "Meta-analysis of Prospective Cohort Studies Evaluating the Association of Saturated Fat with Cardiovascular Disease." *American Journal of Clinical Nutrition* 91 (3): 535–546. doi:10.3945/ajcn.2009.27725

Stubbs, R. J., and C. G. Harbron. 1996. "Covert Manipulation of the Ratio of Medium- to Long-Chain Triglycerides in Isoenergetically Dense Diets: Effect on Food Intake in Ad Libitum Feeding Men." *International Journal of Obesity and Related Metabolic Disorders* 20 (5): 435–444.

Turner, N., K. Hariharan, J. TidAng, G. Frangioudakis, S. M. Beale, L. E. Wright, X. Y. Zeng, et al. 2009. "Enhancement of Muscle Mitochondrial Oxidative Capacity and Alterations in Insulin Action Are Lipid Species Dependent: Potent Tissue-Specific Effects of Medium-Chain Fatty Acids." *Diabetes* 58 (11): 2547–2554. doi:10.2337/db09-0784

Vander Wal, Jillon S., Jorene M. Marth, Pramod Khosla, K.-L. Catherine Jen, and Nikhil V. Dhurandhar. 2005. "Short-Term Effect of Eggs on Satiety in Overweight and Obese Subjects." *Journal of the American College of Nutrition* 24 (6): 510–515. doi:10.1080/07315724.2005.10719497

Wakhloo, A. K., J. Beyer, C. Diederich, and G. Schulz. 1984. "Effect of Dietary Fat on Blood Sugar Levels and Insulin Consumption After Intake of Various Carbohydrate Carriers in Type I Diabetics on the Artificial Pancreas." *DMW—Deutsche Medizinische Wochenschrift* 109 (42): 1589–1594. doi:10.1055/s-2008-1069418

Wien, Michelle, Ella Haddad, Keiji Oda, and Joan Sabaté. 2013. "A Randomized 3X3 Crossover Study to Evaluate the Effect of Hass Avocado Intake on Postingestive Satiety, Glucose and Insulin Levels, and Subsequent Energy Intake in Overweight Adults." *Nutrition Journal* 12 (1). doi:10.1186/1475-2891-12-155

Yamagishi, Kazumasa, Hiroyasu Iso, Hiroshi Yatsuya, Naohito Tanabe, Chigusa Date, Shogo Kikuchi, Akio Yamamoto, et al. 2010. "Dietary Intake of Saturated Fatty Acids and Mortality from Cardiovascular Disease in Japanese: The Japan Collaborative Cohort Study for Evaluation of Cancer Risk (JACC) Study." *American Journal of Clinical Nutrition* 92 (4): 759–765. doi:10.3945/ajcn.2009.29146

Zomer, Ella, Alice Owen, Dianna J. Magliano, Danny Liew, and Christopher M. Reid. 2012. "The Effectiveness and Cost Effectiveness of Dark Chocolate Consumption as Prevention Therapy in People at High Risk of Cardiovascular Disease: Best Case Scenario Analysis Using a Markov Model." *BMJ* 344: e3657. doi:10.1136/bmj.e3657

Rule #5: Watch the Sugar

Abou-Donia, Mohamed B., Eman M. El-Masry, Ali A. Abdel-Rahman, Roger E. McLendon, and Susan S. Schiffman. 2008. "Splenda Alters Gut Microflora and Increases Intestinal P-Glycoprotein and Cytochrome P-450 in Male Rats." *Journal of Toxicology and Environmental Health, Part A* 71 (21): 1415–1429. doi:10.1080/15287390802328630

Avena, Nicole M., Pedro Rada, and Bartley G. Hoebel. 2008. "Evidence for Sugar Addiction: Behavioral and Neurochemical Effects of Intermittent, Excessive

Sugar Intake." *Neuroscience & Biobehavioral Reviews* 32 (1): 20–39. doi:10.1016/j. neubiorev.2007.04.019

Davidson, Terry L., Ashley A. Martin, Kiely Clark, and Susan E. Swithers. 2011. "Intake of High-Intensity Sweeteners Alters the Ability of Sweet Taste to Signal Caloric Consequences: Implications for the Learned Control of Energy and Body Weight Regulation." *Quarterly Journal of Experimental Psychology* 64 (7): 1430–1441. doi:10.1080/17470218.2011.552729

Fried, Susan K., and Salome R. Rao. 2003. "Sugars, Hypertriglyceridemia, and Cardiovascular Disease." *American Journal of Clinical Nutrition* 78 (4): 8735–8805.

Howard, Barbara V., and Judith Wylie-Rosett. 2002. "Sugar and Cardiovascular Disease: A Statement for Healthcare Professionals from the Committee on Nutrition of the Council on Nutrition, Physical Activity, and Metabolism of the American Heart Association." *Circulation* 106 (4): 523–527. doi:10.1161/01. cir.0000019552.77778.04

Schiller, Jeannine S., Jacqueline W. Lucas, Brian W. Ward, and Jennifer A. Peregoy. 2012. "Summary Health Statistics for U.S. Adults: National Health Interview Survey, 2010." National Center for Health Statistics. *Vital and Health Statistics* 10 (252). http://www.cdc.gov/nchs/data/series/sr_10/sr10_252.pdf

Vyas, Ankur, Linda Rubenstein, Jennifer Robinson, Rebecca A. Seguin, Mara Z. Vitolins, Rasa Kazlauskaite, James M. Shikany, et al. 2014. "Diet Drink Consumption and the Risk of Cardiovascular Events: A Report from the Women's Health Initiative." *Journal of General Internal Medicine* 30 (4): 462–468. doi:10.1007/s11606-014-3098-0

Rule #7: Supplement Smartly

Fiber Supplement

Brennan, Charles. 2008. Review of *Dietary Fibre: Components and Functions*, edited by Hannu Salovaara, Fred Gates, and Maija Tenkanen. *Starch/Stärke* 60 (3–4): 209–209. doi:10.1002/star.200890016

Dana, Sheila. 2006. "A Randomized, Double-Blind, Placebo-Controlled Clinical Study Demonstrates Slendesta Potato Protein Extract Is a Safe and Effective Tool for Promoting Weight Reduction." *Kemin Health Technical Literature*, KBB-017-044.

Dana, Sheila, Michael Louie, and Jiang Hu. 2006. "Slendesta Potato Extract Promotes Satiety in Healthy Human Subjects: Iowa State University Study." *Kemin Health Technical Literature*, KHBB-017-050.

Hira, Tohru, Asuka Ikee, Yuka Kishimoto, Sumiko Kanahori, and Hiroshi Hara. 2015. "Resistant Maltodextrin Promotes Fasting Glucagon-Like Peptide-1

Secretion and Production Together with Glucose Tolerance in Rats." *British Journal of Nutrition* 114 (01): 34–42. doi:10.1017/s0007114514004322

Hu, Jiang. 2013. "GRAS Status for Slendesta Potato Extract." *Kemin Health Technical Literature*, KHBB-017-071.

Kishimoto, Yuka, Hiroshi Oga, Hiroyuki Tagami, Kazuhiro Okuma, and Dennis T. Gordon. 2007. "Suppressive Effect of Resistant Maltodextrin on Postprandial Blood Triacylglycerol Elevation." *European Journal of Nutrition* 46 (3): 133–138. doi:10.1007/s00394-007-0643-1

Kishimoto, Yuka, Yuko Yoshikawa, Shoko Miyazato, Hiroshi Oga, Takako Yamada, Hiroyuki Tagami, Chieko Hashizume, et al. 2009. "Effect of Resistant Malto-dextrin on Digestion and Absorption of Lipids." *Journal of Health Science* 55 (5): 838–844. doi:10.1248/jhs.55.838

Livesey, G., and H. Tagami. 2008. "Interventions to Lower the Glycemic Response to Carbohydrate Foods with a Low-Viscosity Fiber (Resistant Maltodextrin): Meta-analysis of Randomized Controlled Trials." *American Journal of Clinical Nutrition* 89 (1): 114–125. doi:10.3945/ajcn.26842

Ye, Zhong, Visalakshi Arumugam, Esther Haugabrooks, Patricia Williamson, and Suzanne Hendrich. 2015. "Soluble Dietary Fiber (Fibersol-2) Decreased Hunger and Increased Satiety Hormones in Humans When Ingested with a Meal." *Nutrition Research* 35 (5): 393–400. doi:10.1016/j.nutres.2015.03.004

Omega-3 Fatty Acids

Bernstein, Adam M., Eric L. Ding, Walter C. Willett, and Eric B. Rimm. 2011. "A Meta-analysis Shows That Docosahexaenoic Acid from Algal Oil Reduces Serum Triglycerides and Increases HDL-Cholesterol and LDL-Cholesterol in Persons Without Coronary Heart Disease." *Journal of Nutrition* 142 (1): 99–104. doi:10.3945/jn.111.148973

Fotuhi, Majid, Payam Mohassel, and Kristine Yaffe. 2009. "Fish Consumption, Long-Chain Omega-3 Fatty Acids and Risk of Cognitive Decline or Alzheimer Disease: A Complex Association." *Nature Reviews Neurology* 5 (3): 140–152. doi:10.1038/ncpneuro1044

Hansen, Anita L., Lisabeth Dahl, Gina Olson, David Thorton, Ingvild E. Graff, Livar Frøyland, Julian F. Thayer, et al. 2014. "Fish Consumption, Sleep, Daily Functioning, and Heart Rate Variability." *Journal of Clinical Sleep Medicine* 10 (5): 567–575.

Jazayeri, Shima, Mehdi Tehrani-Doost, Seyed A. Keshavarz, Mostafa Hosseini, Abolghassem Djazayery, Homayoun Amini, Mahmoud Jalali, et al. 2008. "Comparison of Therapeutic Effects of Omega-3 Fatty Acid Eicosapentaenoic Acid and Fluoxetine, Separately and in Combination, in Major Depressive Disorder." *Australian and New Zealand Journal of Psychiatry* 42 (3): 192–198.

Mohajeri, M. Hasan, Barbara Troesch, and Peter Weber. 2015. "Inadequate Supply of Vitamins and DHA in the Elderly: Implications for Brain Aging and Alzheimer-Type Dementia." *Nutrition* 31 (2): 261–275. doi:10.1016/j.nut.2014.06.016

Morris, Martha Clare, Denis A. Evans, Christine C. Tangney, Julia L. Bienias, and Robert S. Wilson. 2005. "Fish Consumption and Cognitive Decline with Age in a Large Community Study." *Archives of Neurology* 62 (12): 1849. doi:10.1001/archneur.62.12.noc50161

Peuhkuri, Katri, Nora Sihvola, and Riitta Korpela. 2012. "Dietary Factors and Fluctuating Levels of Melatonin." *Food & Nutrition Research* 56 (1): 17252. doi:10.3402/fnr.v56i0.17252

Ramel, Alfons, J. Alfredo Martinez, Mairead Kiely, Narcisa M. Bandarra, and Inga Thorsdottir. 2010. "Moderate Consumption of Fatty Fish Reduces Diastolic Blood Pressure in Overweight and Obese European Young Adults During Energy Restriction." *Nutrition* 26 (2): 168–174. doi:10.1016/j.nut.2009.04.002

Shidfar, F., A. Keshavarz, S. Hosseyni, A. Ameri, and S. Yarahmadi. 2008. "Effects of Omega-3 Fatty Acid Supplements on Serum Lipids, Apolipoproteins and Malondialdehyde in Type 2 Diabetes Patients." *Eastern Mediterranean Health Journal* 14 (2): 305–313.

The New Multivitamin

Adela, Ramu, Roshan M. Borkar, Murali Mohan Bhandi, Gayatri Vishwakarma, P. Naveen Chander Reddy, R. Srinivas, and Sanjay K. Banerjee. 2016. "Lower Vitamin D Metabolites Levels Were Associated with Increased Coronary Artery Diseases in Type 2 Diabetes Patients in India." *Scientific Reports* 6: 37593. doi:10.1038/srep37593

Beard, Jeremy A., Allison Bearden, and Rob Striker. 2011. "Vitamin D and the Anti-viral State." *Journal of Clinical Virology* 50 (3): 194–200.

Giovannucci, Edward, Yan Liu, Bruce W. Hollis, and Eric B. Rimm. 2017. "25-Hydroxyvitamin D and Risk of Myocardial Infarction in Men: A Prospective Study." *Archives of Internal Medicine* 168 (11): 1174–1180. doi:10.1001/archinte.168.11.1174

Rosanoff, Andrea, Connie M. Weaver, and Robert K. Rude. 2012. "Suboptimal Magnesium Status in the United States: Are the Health Consequences Underestimated?" *Nutrition Reviews* 70 (3): 153–164. doi:10.1111/j.1753-4887.2011.00465.x

Urashima, Mitsuyoshi, Takaaki Segawa, Minoru Okazaki, Mana Kurihara, Yasuyuki Wada, and Hiroyuki Ida. 2010. "Randomized Trial of Vitamin D

Supplementation to Prevent Seasonal Influenza A in Schoolchildren." *American Journal of Clinical Nutrition* 91 (5): 1255–1260. doi:10.3945/ajcn.2009.29094

Wang, Lu, Joann E. Manson, Yiqing Song, and Howard D. Sesso. 2010. "Systematic Review: Vitamin D and Calcium Supplementation in Prevention of Cardiovascular Events." *Annals of Internal Medicine* 152 (5): 315–323. doi:10.7326/0003-4819-152-5-201003020-00010

Probiotic

Finegold, Sydney M., Zhaoping Li, Paula H. Summanen, Julia Downes, Gail Thames, Karen Corbett, Scot Dowd, et al. 2014. "Xylooligosaccharide Increases Bifidobacteria but Not Lactobacilli in Human Gut Microbiota." *Food & Function* 5 (3): 436–445. doi:10.1039/c3fo60348b

Gao, Zhanguo, Jun Yin, Jin Zhang, Robert E. Ward, Roy J. Martin, Michael Lefevre, William T. Cefalu, et al. 2009. "Butyrate Improves Insulin Sensitivity and Increases Energy Expenditure in Mice." *Diabetes* 58 (7): 1509–1517. doi:10.2337/db08-1637

Lin, Hua V., Andrea Frassetto, Edward J. Kowalik Jr., Andrea R. Nawrocki, Mofei M. Lu, Jennifer R. Kosinski, James A. Hubert, et al. 2012. "Butyrate and Propionate Protect Against Diet-Induced Obesity and Regulate Gut Hormones via Free Fatty Acid Receptor 3-Independent Mechanisms." *Plos ONE* 7 (4): e35240. doi:10.1371/journal.pone.0035240

Diet Support

Ngondi, Judith L., Blanche C. Etoundi, Christine B. Nyangono, Carl M. F. Mbofung, and Julius E. Oben. 2009. "IGOB131, a Novel Seed Extract of the West African Plant *Irvingia Gabonensis*, Significantly Reduces Body Weight and Improves Metabolic Parameters in Overweight Humans in a Randomized Double-Blind Placebo Controlled Investigation." *Lipids in Health and Disease* 8 (1): 7. doi:10.1186/1476-511x-8-7

Sengupta, Krishanu, Atmatrana T. Mishra, Manikeswar K. Rao, Kadainti V. S. Sarma, Alluri V. Krishnaraju, and Golakoti Trimurtulu. 2012. "Efficacy and Tolerability of a Novel Herbal Formulation for Weight Management on Obese Subjects: A Randomized Double Blind Placebo Controlled Clinical Study." *Lipids in Health and Disease* 11 (1): 122. doi:10.1186/1476-511x-11-122

Sleep Helper

Winkelman, John W., Orfeu M. Buxton, J. Eric Jensen, Kathleen L. Benson, Shawn P. O'Connor, Wei Wang, and Perry F. Renshaw. 2008. "Reduced Brain GABA in Primary Insomnia: Preliminary Data from 4T Proton Magnetic Resonance Spectroscopy (1H-MRS)." *Sleep* 31 (11): 1499–1506. doi:10.1093/sleep/31.11.1499

Extra Magnesium

Golf, Sighart W., S. Bender, and J. Grüttner. 1998. "On the Significance of Magnesium in Extreme Physical Stress." *Cardiovascular Drugs and Therapy* 12 (2): 197–202.

Setaro, Luciana, Paulo Roberto Santos-Silva, Eduardo Yoshio Nakano, Cristiane Hermes Sales, Newton Nunes, Júlia Maria Greve, and Célia Colli. 2013. "Magnesium Status and the Physical Performance of Volleyball Players: Effects of Magnesium Supplementation." *Journal of Sports Sciences* 32 (5): 438–445. doi:10.1080/02640414.2013.828847

Blue Light Protection: Lutein and Zeaxanthin

Juturu, Vijaya, James P. Bowman, Nicole T. Stringham, and James M. Stringham. 2016. "Bioavailability of Lutein/Zeaxanthin Isomers and Macular Pigment Optical Density Response to Macular Carotenoid Supplementation: A Randomized Double Blind Placebo Controlled Study." *New Frontiers in Ophthalmology* 2 (4). doi:10.15761/nfo.1000132

Stringham, James M., Kevin J. O'Brien, and Nicole T. Stringham. 2016. "Macular Carotenoid Supplementation Improves Disability Glare Performance and Dynamics of Photostress Recovery." *Eye and Vision* 3: 30. doi:10.1186/s40662-016-0060-8

Stringham, James M., and Nicole T. Stringham. 2016. "Serum and Retinal Responses to Three Different Doses of Macular Carotenoids over 12 Weeks of Supplementation." *Experimental Eye Research* 151: 1–8. doi:10.1016/j.exer.2016.07.005

Rule #8: Get Some Sleep

Afaghi, Ahmad, Helen O'Connor, and Chin Moi Chow. 2007. "High-Glycemic-Index Carbohydrate Meals Shorten Sleep Onset." *American Journal of Clinical Nutrition* 85 (2): 426–430.

Ayas, Najib T., David P. White, Wael K. Al-Delaimy, JoAnne E. Manson, Meir J. Stampfer, Frank E. Speizer, Sanjay Patel, et al. 2003. "A Prospective Study of Self-Reported Sleep Duration and Incident Diabetes in Women." *Diabetes Care* 26 (2): 380–384. doi:10.2337/diacare.26.2.380

Broussard, Josiane L., David A. Ehrmann, Eve Van Cauter, Esra Tasali, and Matthew J. Brady. 2012. "Impaired Insulin Signaling in Human Adipocytes After

Experimental Sleep Restriction." *Annals of Internal Medicine* 157 (8): 549–557. doi:10.7326/0003-4819-157-8-201210160-00005

Cappuccio, Francesco P., Frances M. Taggart, Ngianga-Bakwin Kandala, Andrew Currie, Ed Peile, Saverio Stranges, and Michelle A. Miller. 2008. "Meta-analysis of Short Sleep Duration and Obesity in Children and Adults." *Sleep* 31 (5): 619–626.

Greer, Stephanie M., Andrea N. Goldstein, and Matthew P. Walker. 2013. "The Impact of Sleep Deprivation on Food Desire in the Human Brain." *Nature Communications* 4: 2259.

St-Onge, Marie-Pierre, Amy L. Roberts, Jinya Chen, Michael Kelleman, Majella O'Keeffe, Arindam RoyChoudhury, and Peter J. H. Jones. 2011. "Short Sleep Duration Increases Energy Intakes but Does Not Change Energy Expenditure in Normal-Weight Individuals." *American Journal of Clinical Nutrition* 94 (2): 410–416. doi:10.3945/ajcn.111.013904

Taheri, Shahrad, Ling Lin, Terry Young, and Emmanuel Mignot. 2004. "Short Sleep Duration Is Associated with Reduced Leptin, Elevated Ghrelin, and Increased Body Mass Index." *PLoS Medicine* 1 (3): 210–217.

Rule #9: Drink Water

Ericson, John. July 3, 2017. "75% of Americans May Suffer from Chronic Dehydration, According to Doctors." *Medical Daily*. http://www.medicaldaily.com/75-americans-may-suffer-chronic-dehydration-according-doctors-247393

Madjd, Ameneh, Moira A. Taylor, Alireza Delavari, Reza Malekzadeh, Ian A. Macdonald, and Hamid R. Farshchi. 2015. "Effects on Weight Loss in Adults of Replacing Diet Beverages with Water During a Hypoenergetic Diet: A Randomized, 24-Wk Clinical Trial." *American Journal of Clinical Nutrition* 102 (6): 1305–1312. doi:10.3945/ajcn.115.109397

Parretti, Helen M., Paul Aveyard, Andrew Blannin, Susan J. Clifford, Sarah J. Coleman, Andrea Roalfe, and Amanda J. Daley. 2015. "Efficacy of Water Preloading Before Main Meals as a Strategy for Weight Loss in Primary Care Patients with Obesity: RCT." *Obesity* 23 (9): 1785–1791. doi:10.1002/oby.21167

Roussel, Ronan, Léopold Fezeu, Nadine Bouby, Beverly Balkau, Olivier Lantieri, François Alhenc-Gelas, Michel Marre, et al. 2011. "Low Water Intake and Risk for New-Onset Hyperglycemia." *Diabetes Care* 34 (12): 2551–2554. doi:10.2337/dc11-0652

Stookey, Jodi D., Florence Constant, Barry M. Popkin, and Christopher D. Gardner. 2008. "Drinking Water Is Associated with Weight Loss in Overweight Dieting Women Independent of Diet and Activity." *Obesity* 16 (11): 2481–2488. doi:10.1038/oby.2008.409

Rule #10: Exercise

Little, Jonathan P., Jenna B. Gillen, Michael E. Percival, Adeel Safdar, Mark A. Tarnopolsky, Zubin Punthakee, Mary E. Jung, et al. 2011. "Low-Volume High-Intensity Interval Training Reduces Hyperglycemia and Increases Muscle Mitochondrial Capacity in Patients with Type 2 Diabetes." *Journal of Applied Physiology* 111 (6): 1554–1560. doi:10.1152/japplphysiol.00921.2011

Ross, Robert, Robert Hudson, Paula J. Stotz, and Miu Lam. 2015. "Effects of Exercise Amount and Intensity on Abdominal Obesity and Glucose Tolerance in Obese Adults." *Annals of Internal Medicine* 162 (5): 325–334. doi:10.7326/m14-1189

Index

Acknowledgments

I T TOOK A VILLAGE to make this book happen and I'm so grateful for each person who was involved.

Dan Mandel, my agent with the patience of a saint, thank you for believing in me from the start so many years ago.

Naomi Whittel, your ideas always push me out of my comfort zone but always into something amazing—I can't thank you enough for all the opportunities.

It's been such an amazing experience working with the BenBella team: Glenn Yeffeth, Adrienne Lang, Sarah Avinger, Monica Lowry, Heather Butterfield, Jennifer Canzoneri, and Rachel Phares. Leah Wilson, I never thought editing could be such a fun and positive experience—thank you for your positivity and great ideas. Rachel Holtzman, thank you for making me a better writer and for your amazing attention to detail.

I thank my amazing team at B Nutritious, Claire Shorenstein and Shane Macintyre. Your hard work and contributions to this book are beyond appreciated.

Jennifer Fisherman Ruff, you really are the best publicist ever. Thank you for your friendship in addition to everything else you do.

Jennifer Cooper and Rob Maru, I'm constantly in awe of you. Your wisdom is incredibly intimidating but in a good way!

Thank you to Niki Simoneaux, Carrieanne Reichardt, Mari Campbell, Carol Goldstein, and all my Diet Detox testers.

I'm grateful to the Fhitting Room team: Kari Saitowitz, Sloan Smith, and the fabulous trainers who contributed to the exercise chapter and kick my butt on a regular basis—Daury Dross, Simon Lawson, Dara Theodore, Ben Wegman, Eric Salvador, Lacee Lazoff, Mark Ribeiro, and Mat Forzaglia.

Helen Rodbell, I'm incredibly lucky to have you as my grandmother.

David and Mia Alpert, you're my voices of reason, laughter, and inappropriate humor.

I thank my parents, Gerry and Hank. Your support literally holds me up. I'm a lucky daughter.

To my husband, Todd, I love you and our crazy life together. Thank you for loving me.

My beautiful daughters: Emma and Ryder, you both are my reason for waking up each day—I love you and am so proud to be your mom.

About the Author

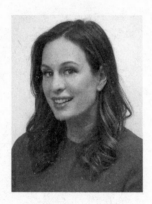

Brooke Alpert, MS, RD, CDN, is a nationally recognized nutrition expert and bestselling author. She is the founder of B Nutritious (www.b-nutritious.com), a private nutrition counseling and consulting practice in New York City.

Brooke's expertise and nutrition knowledge has lead her to be regularly featured on national television, including on *The Dr. Oz Show*, *TODAY*, *Access Hollywood*, and more. She was named one of the new up-and-coming stars in the beauty and health field in *W Magazine* and has been quoted and featured extensively in both national and international magazines, including *PEOPLE*, *Shape*, *Glamour*, *Town & Country*, *Tatler*, and more.

Brooke received her Masters of Science at New York University and completed her training at Mt. Sinai Hospital in affiliation with New York University.

Brooke's previous books include *The Sugar Detox: Lose Weight, Feel Great and Look Years Younger* (Da Capo, 2013) and *Healthy Eating During Pregnancy* (Kyle Books, 2011).

She resides in New York City with her husband and their two daughters.